Table of Contents

Section 1

Introduction

First of all I'd like to say thank you for putting your faith in me and picking up this book.

Over the course of this book you're going to discover how you can lose weight in a fast and permanent, safe and effective way. Not only that but you'll become physically fitter, feel better, look healthier and it will last you for the rest of your life.

I am confident I can do this for you! How do I know? Because as a personal trainer I have already helped hundreds of people achieve this same level of success.

So who is this book for? This book is for the everyday guy or girl who wants to lose weight. It doesn't matter what you have tried in the past, or how many times you have already failed. By putting what you learn in this book into action, you will lose weight. It's as simple as that. By modifying your lifestyle you'll be able to keep the weight off for the rest of your life and live with all the benefits listed above.

So who am I and what are my credentials? My name is James Driver; I have a master's degree in Sport and Exercise Science from Leeds Metropolitan University, England. Leeds Met is one of the UK's specialist institutions in the field. I have worked as a personal trainer for around 12 years. I have helped many hundreds of people achieve their dream figures, including people who had written themselves off. As you may have seen from the other books I have written, I am a professional in the field of healthy living and health and fitness. My book entitled *HIIT – High Intensity Interval Training Explained* is an Amazon best seller and we will be looking at HIIT in this book too as it's my belief that HIIT is the single most effective weight loss method in existence. I hope my credentials speak for themselves.

It is within everyone to look exactly how they would like to, providing the work and effort are put in. However, as we all know, there are right ways and wrong ways about losing weight. Some methods have great success at first and then the results trail off after a couple of weeks. Clearly this is not beneficial for long or even short term weight loss. Some weight loss methods have great success yet are detrimental to the individual's health, ditto this is not good either. Then there are some weight loss strategies that work, they work on an on-going basis and the results are permanent. This is what we should be a ming for and yes, this will happen for you for making the investment in this book.

However, before you embark on the journey for weight loss, you have to acknowledge that simply buying books isn't enough. You have to be willing to put the time and effort in as well. As the old saying goes, you get out what you put in!

Let me clarify also by saying that most "fast weight loss" guides or advice you hear and read about will not be healthy. Fast weight loss in most cases is not permanent weight loss (all will be explained). In this book we are going to learn the "fastest" weight loss techniques which are safe and permanent. These are the best methods and you're about to discover them.

Let's begin.

Is It Genetic?

I would speak to many people at the gym who believed they could never be a slim person because they had the *wrong* genetics. They were born fat, they were fat and they would always be fat. Not only that, but their parents were fat, their brothers and sisters are fat and yes, unfortunately they had even also passed the fat gene down to their children.

This is an extremely defeatist attitude!

Just have a look at photos from the war or earlier and take notice of how our ancestors looked just two generations earlier. Were they all fat? No they were not.

Clearly it is modern lifestyle factors that have caused so many people to become overweight and it is modern life that keeps the weight on. So try telling our grandfathers that obesity is genetic.

Having said that though, genetics is of course very powerful! The genetics we were given at our conception do indeed account for 75% of what we can possibly achieve in weight loss and attaining that dream body. However, within the 25% that is environmental, we can do incredible things.

I would say that the 75% will play a large role in just how quickly we can lose weight, how easy we find it as well as many other factors. We can't change our genetics so let's just forget about it, it's irrelevant. The power we do have is within that huge 25% that is environmental and when we do things correctly, such as in what I will explain, then that 25% is all you'll need.

Genetics should never be used as an excuse, especially considering this obesity epidemic is barely even one or two generations old. Our genetics are all imprinted with thousands of generations as lean hunter-gatherers and only one or two as overweight or obese people. With the right stimuli placed on our bodies, we will revert back to our instinctual and encoded somatotypes; that of lean and athletic individuals.

In any case, even if you are severely overweight, who is to say that this 75% number is conspiring and working against you? If you live a poor and sedentary lifestyle, take part in little to no exercise and over indulge on the good life then things will catch up with you eventually no matter how lucky the genetics you were born with.

It's imperative that as overweight individuals, we should never make excuses for our predicament, but instead we need to take responsibility for the situation we are in. By placing the blame on external factors that we can't control, such as the environment or poor genetics, we are robbing ourselves of the power we have within ourselves to make the changes.

Let's make a promise – No more excuses, it's time to commit to making changes.

Why We Are Overweight

Clearly a lot has changed over the last one or two generations which has transformed the west from a healthy and happy civilization into an overweight and unhealthy one. Presently, roughly 1 in every 3 people in the USA is classed as obese. Even more shocking is that this trend is projected to become even worse. Yet more shocking still is that this is likely to begin with our children.

The reason I'm going to mention the following obesity causes is because it's important we all know why we are overweight in the first place. Prevention would have been better than a cure and by changing our lifestyles for the better, we'll be able to lose our weight quicker and easier, not to mention keep it off once we get to where we want to be.

Let's take a look at the lifestyle factors which have contributed to the obesity epidemic:

Fast Food

McDonalds, Wendy's, Pizza Hut...the list goes on. They are delicious and addictive. In fact they are one of the most addictive things on the planet.

It's not just that they are addictive however, the problem is that they are convenient. We work long hours and we don't always have the energy for cooking a nice, healthy meal late at night. So instead we simply go for a tasty fast food take-away. The fact that they are also incredibly cheap to buy does not help either.

Portion Sizes

We will discuss this in detail later on. Portion sizes have a huge effect on our overall weight. It takes a strong person to quit eating when there's still food in front of you, even if you're already full. Unfortunately, your body cannot digest large amounts of food in one go, so a large quantity of your meal will be stored as fat.

Many restaurants, fast food restaurants in particular are competing with their rivals for your business. The place you spend your money will often be the place that heaps up the largest portions on your plate.

Processed Food

Food companies process food in order to take out harmful chemicals and food borne diseases. Processing can also prolong the life of the food too. Unfortunately, processing raw food ingredients such as wheat removes many natural elements such as fibre. As a consequence wheat intolerances are becoming more common. But just as important when it comes to your weight is that it's the fibre that actually adds bulk to the food, thus helping to fill you up. Fibre cannot be digested in the human gut and so is removed as waste. This is why a diet high in fibre is great because you feel full when you eat but you don't pile on the pounds. With less fibre being found in our meals, clearly this is no longer the case in as high a proportion.

Snacking

If done correctly then I'm not against snacking per se. I will explain why you should "snack" and how best to do it later.

However, the problem arises when we have large meals and then snack in between them. This all adds to the calorie count and to our weight. Whenever we go to the gas station or supermarket, there are snacks conveniently located so that we make eye contact with them. It takes a strong person to spot them and ignore them.

Convenience

Society has changed so much that it's actually becoming increasingly difficult to carry out any physical activity at all. In fact, the only way we can do any exercise these days is if we deliberately set out to do it.

I'll explain that a little more - Fifty years ago when we went and did the shopping, we'd have to go to several different shops in order to pick everything up, dashing all around town in the process. These days, everything is kept under one roof. You only need to drive to Walmart or Tesco and you can collect a full week's worth of food in one go with barely any effort on your part. Heck, you can even get your car, travel or household insurance sorted out in the same building.

Even more recently, you don't even need to venture to Walmart or Tesco for your shopping at all. You simply need to logon to the internet and order your food online, it'll even be delivered to your front door. No need to exercise ever again!

On the rare occasion we go to the shopping mall, we always drive, even though we could probably walk there in 30 minutes or under. Once at the mall, we have lifts, elevators or escalators so we don't need to exert ourselves climbing any stairs.

Put simply...Society has made getting any exercise difficult!

If we want to make improvements then obviously we're going to have to buck the trend and change our lifestyles, becoming rebels against the system. We must be different! This will most likely take a huge effort but you'll feel better for it. Later on we'll look at a range of ways you can incorporate physical activity into your everyday lifestyle.

Measuring Weight Loss

This is important! Please don't skip this section simply because you don't think we're yet getting into the fine details. Trust me; the fine details are right here.

You're about to find out one of the biggest reasons why people become disheartened and fail at weight loss and it all has to do with how they measure their results.

First of all, when we embark upon a weight loss program, we should all be taking a variety of base mark readings with which to judge our success. If you don't take any readings prior to starting your journey then how will you know if you're losing weight and becoming healthier?

However, one thing I will never recommend you measure your results by is your weight.

Read that last paragraph again.

But wait a minute; aren't we supposed to be trying to lose weight here? That is true, but in reality, what we would really like to do is to lose *fat*! The two; weight and fat are not necessarily the same thing.

I know for a fact, from working with many hundreds of people as a personal trainer that at least half of all people who embark on a weight loss program, and do it the right way actually *gain* weight when they begin their program. Typically this will correct itself after around three or four weeks when the actual weight will start to drop off.

Now there are two significant things to this. Firstly, imagine starting a weight loss programme and then after three weeks, you weigh yourself to find that you had actually gained weight, or at the very least kept the same weight, you'd be disheartened and quite possibly give up I would expect. This happens more frequently than you could imagine. It's a known fact that 75% of new gym attendees will stop attending the gym after six weeks. Now you know why they get you to sign up for a full year.

Unfortunately, not all people who start going to the gym actually have anybody knowledgeable to tell them why they are gaining weight and why it's not a bad thing. This brings me to my second point.

When you join a gym, most often the new members haven't carried out any exercise for many years. All of a sudden they are becoming very active. This places a huge amount of stress on the body. Living organisms adapt and evolve under stress, this is nature after all. This stress causes our bodies to change to better be able to cope with the new conditions, such as exercise. So what the body actually does is build more muscle. Muscle is heavier than fat, by a long way. So after say three weeks of attending a gym for the first time, the weight you've gained is, and should actually be muscle. This is an extremely positive occurrence for you because fat and energy are metabolised within the muscle, so the more muscle you have, the more you'll be able to burn off the fat and lose the weight, although most of this will come later on.

The problem for those poor unguided people who then go on to weigh themselves several times every week is that they don't realise the weighing scale cannot tell the difference between fat and muscle. It's simply weighing your overall body mass.

This is why you should never use a weighing scale to judge your success when it comes to weight loss, especially during the early stages of a weight loss regime.

Instead, you should take a baseline measurement using the following techniques and then measure again every two to four weeks hence to judge your success:

Waist / Hip Ratio

Actually measuring the circumference of your waist is as simple yet effective a way as any for gaging your progress. It is after all the fat you're wanting rid of, so why not go direct? By performing a simple calculation with the circumference measurements of the waist and hips, you end up with a good idea of how much fat you actually have when compared to what is desirable.

It's important that the same person takes the measurements every time you take the test in order to ensure standardisation. If you're wearing clothes when taking the measurement then always wear the same clothes, or not if that's the case. A soft anthropometric tape is preferred for accuracy.

The waist circumference must obviously be taken at the same position every time you take the test. Therefore you should take the measurement along the circumference at the belly button.

For measuring the hips, find the area of greatest circumference. To do this you can move the tape measure up or down until you find the largest area of circumference.

Take a note of both measurements and put them into the following equation:

Waist (cm/inches) / Hips (cm/inches) =

So for example, a man with a 79cm waist and 86cm hips would have a waist to hips ratio of 0.92. Is this good? Refer to the chart below for where your ratio falls:

Waist to Hip Ratio Chart

Male	Female	Health Risk
0.95 or below	0.80 or below	Low
0.96 - 1.0	0.81 - 0.85	Moderate
1.0 +	0.85 +	High

It's important to realise that obviously desirable ratios differ for men and women due to differing hip sizes and where body fat is typically stored. Men tend to store more fat around their waists, whereas women store it around their hips. The chart is modified accordingly.

Once you've taken your baseline measurement, of course it will be tempting to compare your ratio with that of the chart. However, what you get at baseline really doesn't matter. What matters is that the next time you take your measurement in say four weeks in the future, the ratio is lower. That is how you should be judging your success and by nothing else. You're competing against yourself here and not the rest of society.

BMI

Now I contradict myself a little here. Taking your body mass index (BMI) measurement involves taking your height and your weight and finding the ratio between the two to see if you're a healthy weight for your height.

Now I know I said not to weigh yourself but I make an exception for discovering your BMI. The reason for this is that you will have a good baseline reading of how healthy you are, and then in a year's time you'll be able to see just how far you've come when the number is drastically improved.

Another reason for measuring BMI is that it's important we know where we're starting from. Often, we may think we're obese when in actual fact we're simply overweight, when categorised by the BMI scale.

To calculate your BMI simply divide your body weight in Kg by your height in M^2. For those in America, simply take your weight in lbs and then multiply that number by 703 then divide that number by your height in inches[2].

You are overweight if your BMI equals 25 or above. If it's above 30 then you are classed as obese.

But once again, remember that this is simply a baseline measurement. What really matters is that your BMI reduces the next time you take your reading. In any case, as already stated, you should only take your BMI readings with a pinch of salt in the early stages since it doesn't take into account your actual body composition, being unable to distinguish between muscle, fat or even any excess water or lack thereof you may be holding.

Body Fat

You can get fairly accurate body fat readings by measuring skinfold fat thickness at four sites on the body.

All gyms have skinfold callipers to take measurements and many of the gym staff will be proficient in using them. I would suggest you get the same staff member (assuming you're a member of a gym) to take your reading every time in order to ensure standardisation.

Since this is something you won't be doing yourself, I won't go into the specifics of how the test is taken, but it involves using a pair of callipers to get a skinfold thickness reading on the bicep, tricep, side of the belly and lower back. The readings are then added together to give you a body fat percentage. A good trainer should be able to complete this reading within two minutes.

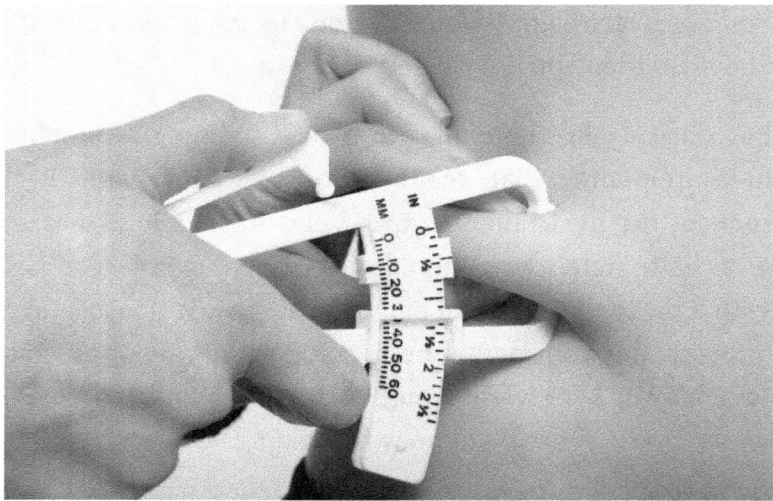

When you have your body fat %, simply make a note of it for the next time you have the test taken.

Summary

- Never judge your success by your weight, especially in the early stages of a weight loss routine.
- Take baseline measurements of waist/hip ratio, BMI and body fat instead of your weight.
- Take measurements every four weeks.

The Fundamentals of Weight Loss

When it comes to losing weight, it all boils down to the following graphical equation:

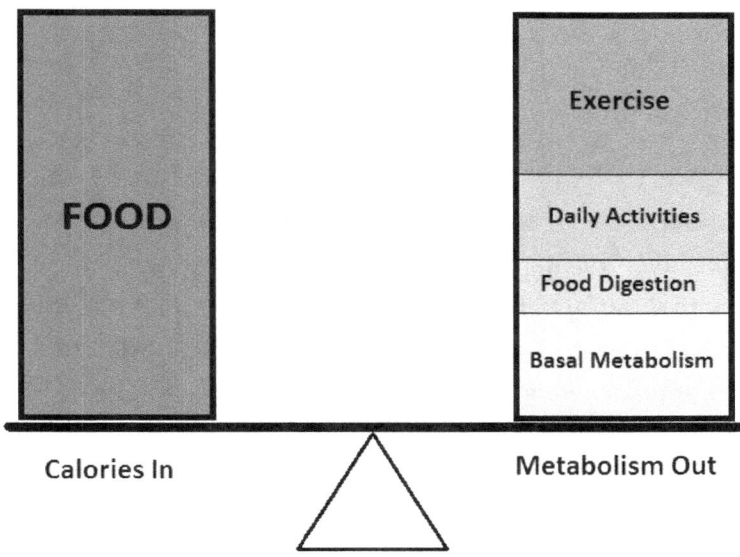

We'll probably find that as this book progresses, my drawings get a little better.

As you can see, if the amount of calories your body metabolises is equal to the calories you take in through food then your weight will stay the same. If you take in more calories than your body metabolises then you will gain weight, it's as simple as that. Then of course if your body metabolises more than you take in in calories then you will lose weight. It really is that straightforward, though of course there are a few caveats here and there which we will get into.

Let's discuss each part of the diagram now:

Calories In - Food

The recommended daily intake of calories for a male is 2500 and for a female 1800.

Be wary of what you read with regards to these calorific amounts being any higher than this. They have been set at this level for many years and you may read in some places that they are higher. This is for reasons of political correctness and there is no room for the PC brigade when it comes to weight loss. I have always preferred the blunt and direct approach to this subject and my clients have always appreciated it. Nature does not give a damn as to political correctness and those people who say that the above daily calorific requirements are any higher really should be ashamed of themselves.

Now you may be tempted to tip the scale on the above drawing over to the right by dieting and taking in less food. This is ok *to an extent* - But please read the following line carefully:

You do not want to cut your recommended daily calorific intake by more than 10%!

The reason many people fail at weight loss is locked inside that line of text above! I'll explain more in a bit.

Metabolism Out – Basal Metabolism

Your basal or basic metabolic rate refers to the amount of calories your body will use simply to function and keep you alive. These are the easy calories we burn while we're sleeping or watching TV. At any one moment there are billions of chemical reactions going on in our bodies and all these reactions use up energy.

From looking at the picture you can see that it is perhaps the joint second largest slice of all metabolism. Did you know that you can actually increase the share and quantity of energy that is burned through basal metabolism, thus increasing the amount of calories you burn while you watch TV (for more on this, see the section on *HIIT*)?

All energy is used within an organelle in our cells. This organelle is called the mitochondria which has been given the nickname of our cell's "powerhouse." All our cells have many mitochondria, however the cells where energy is burned in greater abundance, for example our muscle cells have many more of them. When we exercise, our bodies actually create more mitochondria in order to power the increase in activity. Not only that but the existing mitochondria grow in size too, making them more efficient and powerful.

Because of the increase in number and size of mitochondria in our cells, this helps burn more energy even when we aren't doing anything. Of course this is an incentive to keep exercising and not to give up as greater results come the longer you stick at it.

Metabolism Out – Food Digestion

The calorific expenditure used in food digestion is also known as the Thermic Effect of Food (TEF). TEF is the smallest section of the graphical equation above yet still comprises a considerable amount over the course of the year, it would be wrong not to talk a little about it here.

It is known that all protein intake will be metabolised through TEF to the degree of 30%. This is by no means a small quantity. Fat intake will be metabolised only at 2%, which is next to negligible. So it looks like you're going to have to deal with your fat intake via another method. Carbohydrate TEF comes in at around 15%, which is not unwelcome.

For example, if we eat a piece of chicken (protein) that contains 500 calories, by the time it has been digested, there will only be 350 calories left in our body. If we then eat a jacket potato (carbohydrate) that was the exact same 500 calories, by the time it had been digested, there would be 425 calories left in our body. Finally, if we then eat a piece of lard (fat) that was the same 500 calories (please don't do this) then by the time our body had metabolised it, there would still be 490 calories from the lard left in our body.

There is nothing we can do unfortunately to alter these ratios and make our bodies metabolise more fat on autopilot simply through digestion. Just be aware of the fact that this is one of the reasons why we need to lower our fat intake, since nature gives us no helping hand here.

Metabolism Out – Daily Activities

To lose weight fast, we really need to be increasing our energy expenditure through every day activities. We use up energy all the time, no matter what we are doing, the more strenuous the activity, the more energy we are using.

There are literally thousands of daily activities I could list here, some of the better ones will be listed later on. Things from vacuuming and washing the car to walking to work or doing the shopping all use up energy. Everybody should work on increasing the amount of energy they use through every day activities.

Metabolism Out – Exercise

As you can see from the graphical equation above, exercise is the big one. If you don't exercise, or at least have an active lifestyle through your daily activities then it's unlikely you'll be metabolising enough calories to deal with what you're taking in through food.

Now we are going to go and have a more detailed look at the two most important fundamental elements of weight loss; what you take in through calories and what you metabolise through activity. Remember that if you expend more calories than what you are taking in then you will lose weight.

Section 2

Calories In

Diet

Please read every word of this section carefully as I believe it will alter your entire thought process with regards to nutrition and you'll never "diet" in the same way again.

In order for us to stay happy and healthy, we need to take in adequate amounts of nutrients. These nutrients are as follows:

- Protein
- Carbohydrate
- Fat
- Vitamins
- Minerals
- Water

We get our calories from the first three on that list. As already stated, fully grown men require 2500 calories per day and women require 1800.

1 gram of protein = 4 calories

1 gram of carbohydrate = 4 calories

1 gram of fat = 9 calories

As you can see, in order to lose weight, it's obvious why we need to cut down on our fat intake. Consider also that fat is actually the least satiating of the three, in that fat will fill you up less than protein and carbohydrate even though a single gram of fat contains more than twice the calories of protein or carbs.

Yet again, nature does not help us out when it comes to fat!

Then you also have alcohol - 1 gram contains 7 calories.

Depending on how much you drink, this may or may not be a factor for you. In any case, I would never tell you to give up one of life's great pleasures. Just be aware that a single gram of alcohol contains 7 calories. This amount is actually negligible due to the fact there is very little pure alcohol in any alcoholic drink; at least the drinks that people drink regularly.

In addition fibre can kind of be included as a nutrient. The difference is that fibre cannot be digested by the human gut and therefore cannot be utilised for energy.

1 gram of fibre = 0 calories

By having a diet high in fibre, you are adding a major weight loss tool to your arsenal. Fibre serves to add bulk to your food, filling you up yet not adding to the calorific intake one bit. Remember what I said above about modern food processing removing fibre from our diets? This is not a good thing. In fact it explains why we are eating more and getting larger since what we are eating is not filling us up as much as it used to. Fibre also helps to lower cholesterol which is obviously important in keeping us healthy.

Food processing in wheat for example removes the outer shell which contains the fibre. Therefore a great source of fibre is whole-wheat products where the shell has not been removed. For weight loss, you should begin eating whole-wheat products such as pasta and bread. Other sources of fibre are; brown rice, broccoli, lentils and unprocessed fruit and vegetables.

When buying food, try and buy foods that are as close as possible to their natural state.

Protein

I'm sure you've heard of protein, its functions and uses. But just in case you haven't I'll fill you in now.

Protein is used in the body for growth, maintenance and repair. You will find protein in the building blocks of every single cell in the body as well as in our muscles, skin ligaments, bones, hair, teeth and nails. Protein provides much of the structure to all of these things.

However, in addition to that, protein also makes up all enzymes in the body. Enzymes are used to regulate every single chemical reaction that takes place in your body, billions of them.

Proteins are actually made from smaller components called amino acids. In total there are 20 different amino acids. 12 of these the body can make on its own and 8 of them the body needs to get from the food we take in. The 12 the body can make are called non-essential amino acids, and the 8 that the body cannot make on its own are called essential amino acids.

Please try and understand this as it has great importance later on in this book.

When a non-essential amino acid is in short supply, the body can easily create a new one. However when an essential amino acid is needed, its creation will not be able to take place until it is supplied through nutrition.

So we really need to make sure that our diets are topped up with the 8 essential amino acids. Don't worry; this won't be a problem for the vast majority of people as they are contained in abundance within animal produce; eggs, milk and cheese. Rice, legumes and nuts are also good sources.

Protein is of course used for many important functions in the body, however it is not often and should not often be used in energy production. Protein can indeed be used as a source of energy, to power exercise and your everyday activities, but I'm sure you'd agree, it would be much better if fat was used for this purpose instead. The problem is that for many individuals, the body is using too high a proportion of protein, straight from their muscle cells to power activity, instead of using the abundant fat stores.

Daily protein needs = 10 – 15% of total calorie intake.

You may have read in many places that increasing your protein intake is a positive thing. This is not true for bodybuilders and it's certainly not true for those of us that are trying to lose weight.

In fact, having an excess of protein in the diet can be detrimental for weight loss as taking in more than the 15% requirement will simply cause the body to store the excess as fat.

In addition, there are other health detriments to having a diet too high in protein such as the possibility of kidney damage due to the kidneys not being able to excrete the surplus of protein. In addition, a high level of protein in the bloodstream can lead to an accumulation of ammonia which is toxic to brain cells.

Fat

Despite what you may believe about fat, it is actually essential to our survival and it plays many important functions within the body such as:

- The protection, through insulation of internal organs.
- Protection, through insulation of nerve cells.
- Temperature control.
- Regulation of certain vitamins.
- Growth, development and repair of body tissues. Like protein, fat is used in the walls of our cells.
- Fats in our skin give us radiant complexions and make our hair look healthy and glossy. You can tell when somebody does not have much fat in their diet due to their skin looking dull.
- Energy - Remember that 1 gram of fat will give us 9 kcals (calories) of energy. This equates to 3500 calories for every pound of fat.

Daily fat needs = 30 - 35% of total calorie intake.

The problem is that on average people are taking in more than the 30 - 35% that is recommended to maintain healthy living. In western nations the average fat intake is approaching 40% of total calorie intake. This is clearly what is leading to an obesity problem. This extra 5 – 10% which we are taking in may not sound like a lot, but over the course of the years and especially if we are not carrying out enough exercise, this is the reason why the extra weight piles onto our bodies, silently and without us realising it.

Remember that there are 9 calories per gram of fat, more than twice the amount found in carbs or protein. This means that if your diet is too high in fat, it's going to be over proportionately high in calories too. How will these extra calories be stored? That's correct, as fat!

Now, in the context of weight loss, or more specifically fat loss, we would like to create a situation where our bodies are able to utilise fat as its primary source of energy and not protein or carbohydrate. Read on...

Carbohydrate

If 10% of our calorific intake should be from protein and 30% from fat then that leaves the remaining 60% which should be from carbohydrates.

Daily carbohydrate needs = 60% of total calorie intake.

It's true that carbs do have structural duties to perform in the body, however by far their most important function is to provide energy to the cells.

Before carbs can be used as energy in the body, they have to be converted into glucose. Glucose is the body's energy source of choice because it is extremely abundant and easy to create and metabolise.

It's true that the majority of the body's cells can use mixtures of fat, protein and carbohydrate for energy. However the brain itself is only capable of using glucose for energy which must come from carbohydrates. In actual fact, carbohydrates must always be converted to glucose prior to being used for energy no matter where it is in the body.

There are two types of carbohydrates that you'll find in the diet:

Simple Sugars

Sweet tasting and sticky to the touch; sugar, sweets, jams.

Complex Sugars

More dense; bread, cereals, pasta, rice, potatoes, vegetables.

Both forms of carbs are the same when it comes to calorie counts; they both carry 4 calories to the gram.

The difference comes in their molecular structure:

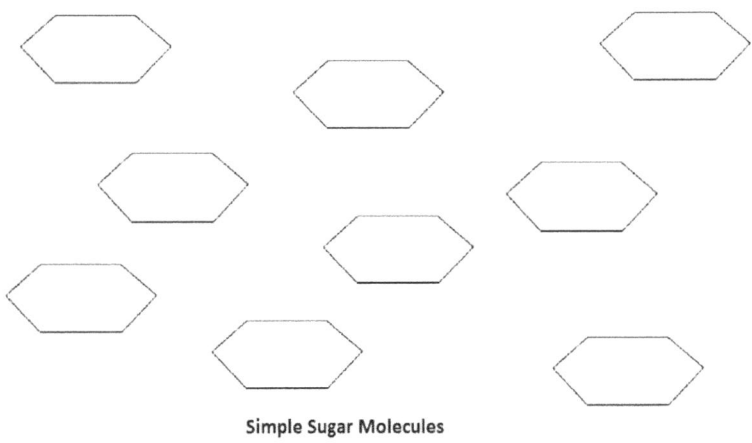

Simple Sugar Molecules

Each molecule is actually one unit of glucose which is ready to be used as energy straight away. Eating carbohydrate in simple sugar form will not fill you up because the molecules are so small.

Now let's take a look at complex sugar molecules:

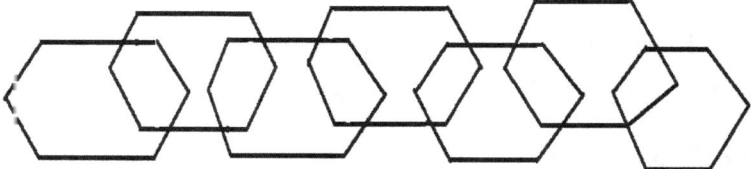

A Complex Sugar Molecule

Ckay, so I lied earlier and my drawings aren't getting better as the book progresses. But as you can see, a single molecule of complex sugars or complex carbs is very large when compared to the simple variety. These serve to fill you up! Not only that but foods which contain these complex sugars also tend to contain fibre in abundance as well.

This complex sugar molecule is actually called glycogen. Glycogen is stored in small quantities in our muscles until we need it, for example when we exercise. Unfortunately the body is unable to store any more than a 6 hour glycogen supply which has large effects on our metabolism which we'll discuss in a bit.

When we eat simple sugars, since they are already in the form the body uses as energy; glucose, the body will try to use it up straight away. This is why many athletes eat sugary snacks prior to a training session or marathon etc. If we eat a lot of sugar in one go and the body can't metabolise it straight away, then the pancreas will dispatch insulin to deal with it. Insulin serves to bind each small sugar molecule together, thus turning them into the longer glycogen chains for use later. However the pancreas can only create small amounts of insulin at a time, so what happens to the excess glucose?

Well glucose is actually toxic when left in the blood for long periods. So when we eat a lot of sugar, this is why we get the energy boost, but then the toxic effect serves to bring us down and make us tired within a very short period of time thereafter. Eventually the excess glucose, instead of being used as energy straight away will instead be converted to yet more fat. The added detriment is that over time, we may become a type II diabetic.

This is why I recommend to you that your diet needs to be as low as possible in simple sugars!

Your diet should instead be high in the complex carbohydrates, which fill you up. In the unlikely event that you do eat too many complex carbohydrate calories, the body actually uses energy to convert them into fat. Thus increasing the energy you spend through food digestion or TEF. Remember when we discussed this earlier? An over consumption of fat to the sum of 300 calories will lead to fat storage in your body of 294 calories. Whereas an over consumption of 300 complex carbohydrate calories will lead to a fat storage of 255 calories. That's quite a big difference! However, due to the large molecular structure of complex carbohydrates and in addition the high fibre content, over indulgence in complex carbohydrates just isn't that easy anyway.

C early for fast weight loss, it is evident why we need to ircrease our intake of complex carbohydrates and dɘcrease our consumption of simple sugars and fat.

Water Intake

We will now backtrack a little bit to talk about the most important nutrient of them all.

Most people know that around 60% of our bodies are water! Its importance to our well-being is unsurpassed by any other nutrient. Some of the many important functions water serves to do are:

- Temperature regulation. When we exercise, water distributes the heat from your working muscles to the skins surface.
- Water is the body's transportation system. It moves everything around your body; vitamins, minerals, nutrients etc. It also removes waste products.
- Every single chemical reaction in your body takes place within water.

Yet what most people aren't aware of is that the vast majority of us are walking around, spending our day to day lives being severely dehydrated the vast majority of the time.

Being dehydrated can cause us some terrible problems such as:

- Fatigue
- Irritability
- Dry skin and rashes

- Rapid heart beat
- Low blood pressure
- Greater susceptibility to illnesses
- Fever
- Headaches
- Brain fog and poor concentration
- Pain in joints
- Poor digestion
- There is also evidence that being dehydrated for a long time can lead to Alzheimer's disease.

A loss of just 2% of our body weight as water will seriously affect our mood and performance. A further loss of 5% can be fatal to us!

Throughout the day, while we eat, sleep, work, exercise or play we lose water continuously. It is estimated that a sedentary person will lose eight cups of water every day simply by living.

A loss of 2% of water, something that happens to us all the time simply by living will slow down our body's chemical reactions. This will of course include our metabolism, lowering our BMR. A 2% loss of water will slow down our energy generation meaning that we're burning less calories by sitting still or carrying out any exercise, we will also feel tired!

To put another number on this, the average human body will lose 2 − 2.5 litres/4 − 5 pints of water at rest, by spending all day watching TV. Are you replacing this water? Of course, as you get up, go to work and exercise, this fluid loss increases significantly. One hour of exercise, intensity and weather dependant could be responsible for a further loss of 2 litres of water.

Therefore, when you become more active, which you will be doing if you follow this book, you will have a water requirement of around 5 litres a day or 8 – 9 pints.

Of course, much of this water will come from your food. Fruit and vegetables contain quite a lot of water and your body is easily able to extract this water. During an average day, your body can probably obtain between 1 and 2 litres of water like this. However, to remain healthy and hydrated, this still leaves a lot of water that you need to take in. Are you taking in this much water?

When I say *water*, I'm not talking about fluid - I'm talking about water! Water contained within soda or fizzy drinks does not count towards your hydration; in fact they count against you! When fluids contain a sugar content above 6% then they actually serve to dehydrate you, since the blood contains 6% sugar. This rules out all fizzy drinks!

Caffeinated drinks such as coffee also count against you. They work to actually speed up the water loss from your body. Most fruit juices, though healthy, also contain a large quantity of sugar which will speed up water loss. I'm not saying you can't have any of these things, but you should always ensure you take in an extra quantity of water for all coffee or sugary drinks you take in.

You should also not use your thirst as an indicator of how hydrated/dehydrated you are! This is because thirst is a physiological response to dehydration, so if you feel thirsty, you are already dehydrated.

The best thing you can do therefore is to drink small amounts of water often throughout the day. Try not to ever feel thirsty! This is by far the best way of handling this.

However, when it comes to weight loss, there are a few important reasons why we should be drinking plenty of water:

- Research has shown that people who drink 8 – 12 glasses of water a day have higher metabolisms than those who drink only four glasses or less. One study showed you can increase your metabolic rate by 30% over the next 30 – 40 minutes simply by drinking a glass of water. This is because your body is working to heat up the water to your core temperature. This could transpire to an extra 17000 Kcals a year simply by increasing your water intake by 1.5 litres a day, which is all the study went up to. Let's be very conservative and half that amount and say 8500 fat calories. This means that 950 grams of fat a year would be lost. Let's call it 1Kg of lost fat in a year or 2.2 lbs simply by increasing your water intake.
- Drinking nice cold water also helps you to feel fuller, so you end up eating less but more

importantly you'll be less tempted to over indulge. We've already spoken briefly about not eating large quantities; water with your meals is a partial cure for this. The American Dietetic Association has also found in a study that people who drank water prior to a meal actually ate 75 Kcal less during the meal. This adds up to a lot over the course of a year.

- Water is known to help the speedy digestion of your food, decreasing the amount you store as fat.

Please don't underestimate the power of drinking lots of water for your weight loss, it will help you significantly. It is a large part of the total weight loss puzzle that you should be incorporating into your arsenal.

Energy for Weight Loss

I'll clarify here that for the body to use carbohydrates for energy, the carbs first need to be broken down into the smaller glucose units. For fat to be used as energy, the fat molecules need to be broken down into smaller units called fatty acids. For protein to be used as energy they need to be broken back down into their component amino acids.

At any one time, the body is actually using all three nutrients for energy albeit in different proportions depending on what you're doing.

The body finds it far easier and far preferential to use glucose through carbohydrate as energy, it's just the way nature is I'm afraid. Although, for weight loss, we really need to create a condition within our bodies so that it prefers to use fat as it's number 1 energy source or at least to use a greater proportion of fat when compared to carbohydrates. Protein is used only as an emergency energy supply, as it is locked in your muscles. Protein tends to be used when you're starving and is clearly the opposite of what we're trying to achieve.

Our muscles need a supply of energy in order to contract; this energy comes in the form of a chemical called Adenosine Triphosphate (ATP). ATP is extremely high in energy.

Because ATP is so very high in energy, it cannot actually be stored in the muscles, or anywhere else for that matter, but instead must be made to order and then used instantly. A safer, more stable and less energetic chemical however can be stored safely in the muscles, it is very similar to ATP. Adenosine Diphosphate (ADP) is stored in our muscles along with stray single phosphate molecules. Energy is created when the stray phosphates are connected to the ADP to form ATP. However, they can only do this when there is fuel! This fuel is carbohydrate, fat and protein. These three are used in different proportions depending on the intensity of the activity being performed and also our present levels of glycogen in the blood – remember that our bodies can store a six hour supply of glycogen before it becomes depleted.

However, in addition to carbs, fat and protein, there is also a fourth energy source compound which doesn't come direct from food. This is called Creatine Phosphate (CP)! CP is used to create ATP only under the most intense circumstances such as a 100% all-out effort such as sprinting. CP stores run out within ten seconds which explains why you can't sprint for longer than that amount of time, even after many years of training.

Obviously the fat and carbohydrate which are used to create ATP or energy comes from our stored food supply. Remember that carbs are stored in glycogen form, long chains of glucose connected together and stored in the liver and muscles. Fat on the other hand cannot really be stored in the muscle, not in large amounts anyway but is instead stored all over the place; you know this right?

When you exercise and the body needs to utilise fat for energy, the body will take it from wherever it can get it from. Anywhere and everywhere! Know this now, that if you have fat in one place that you're trying to get rid of, the body can't target fat for removal in any one place, it'll take the fat from everywhere all at once. However, because men have more fat around their bellies and women keep more of it around their hips; this is where the body will naturally take it from since this is where it is most abundant. No matter what you may hear or read, "spot reductions" or losing weight in one area is not something that you can have any control over! Your body will take fat from wherever it can grab it from and, when it needs it!

As I've already said, carbohydrate and fat will very rarely be utilized for energy alone, but will be used together in varying proportions depending on your present activity levels.

High intensity, short duration exercises will depend mainly on carbohydrate for energy since glucose is more easily used to create ATP and the body has an urgent need of fast created energy at high intensities. In addition high intensity exercises, or anaerobic exercises meaning in the absence of oxygen cannot be powered using fat as fat cannot be metabolised without the use of oxygen. Oxygen is not used anaerobically.

However, when the intensity drops, a greater proportion of fat is used for energy as opposed to carbohydrate. This is aerobic activity and is used in the vast majority of circumstances from sleeping and watching TV all the way up to exercise at around 80 – 85% of your maximal heart rate, when the activity becomes anaerobic and you get a build-up of lactic acid.

The higher the intensity, the lower the proportion of fat utilisation even if the exercise remains aerobic!

However...

It is a fact that no matter how low in intensity or how aerobic the activity or exercise is, the human body can't burn fat alone! Fat can only be used for energy in conjunction with carbohydrate!

Please read that last paragraph again.

Energy Usage Levels With High Glycogen Supply

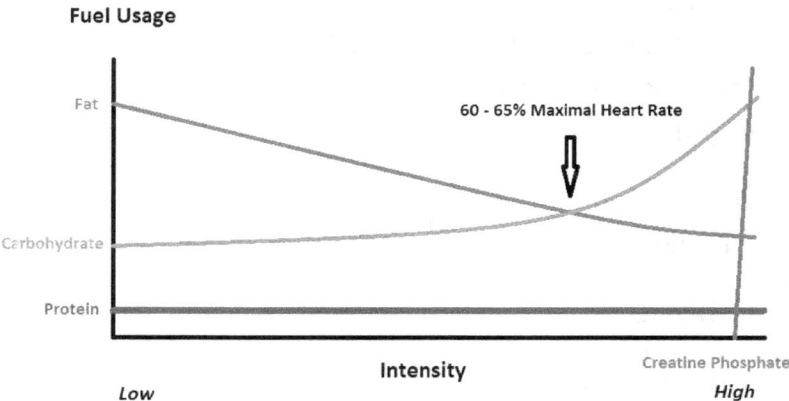

Please study the above graph.

As you can see, fat utilisation is higher at the lower intensities and declines as the activity becomes more intense. There is though a caveat to this rule that I will explain later on, why I still advocate for higher intensity activities for increased fat burning. You will find out why later on and it will change your entire mind set to exercise.

Carbohydrate usage is low at first and becomes the main energy source at around the level of 60 – 65% of maximal heart rate.

Protein usage remains constantly low which is a good thing. Creatine phosphate kicks in once the intensity reaches 95% or above.

How long does your body's glycogen supply last for?

If you remain sedentary then it will last for around six hours. However, when you perform physical activity, this time reduces. This has large implications for fat loss!

For the vast majority of people, when they exercise, even under low intensities of say 60% of their maximal heart rate (a brisk paced walk) the ratio of fat to carbohydrate used will most likely be around 50:50.

You should know that the more you train, the more this ratio improves in favour of fat burning as your body becomes more efficient at using fat as its primary source of fuel.

While we go about our daily business, doing the shopping, preparing dinner or sitting at our desks working, our bodies will be using primarily fat as a fuel source, but of course also a lot of carbohydrate too.

But just to clarify, the efficient and effective utilisation of fat as a fuel source to power your body depends greatly on maintaining an adequate glycogen store within your muscles which in turn of course depends on you maintaining an adequate daily supply of carbohydrate. This is because as you know, our body's ability to actually store carbohydrate is limited to 6 hours maximum.

So what happens when your body runs out of carbohydrate, glycogen supply? Well your body still has fat, but it can no longer use this as energy in any great quantity, so where else can your body get the fuel from to power your ever decreasing activity and energy levels?

That's right, from your protein stores, which can only come from your lean muscle! So in effect your body is cannibalising itself when you starve to power activity. Remind yourself exactly where fat is burned in your body - Where exactly? That's right, in your muscles. So when you lose muscle mass due to starvation, or simply from running out of your six hour glycogen supply, your body is in fact losing its potential to burn fat in the future! This clearly has great implications for weight loss regimes.

Energy Usage Levels With No Glycogen Supply

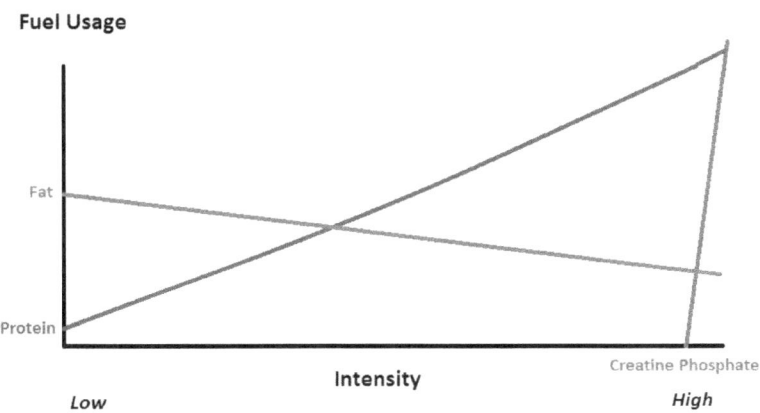

In this graph you can see how things change with no glycogen supply. If you take away the carbohydrates, because the person to whom this graph belongs has not eaten anything since yesterday's evening meal, having skipped breakfast etc then you can see that protein comes to the front as the dominant energy source. This happens soon too, at a lower intensity. If you go for a work out with no glycogen supply, the amount of protein used to supply the activity increases further as the amount of fat used decreases rapidly.

Remember that protein should not be used to supply energy, only in emergencies! Much better to keep topped up with complex carbohydrates which will also boost our fat usage!

If you habitually skip lunch and then go to the gym straight after work, you may want to rethink your routine.

Let's clarify again. Having a 30 minute run on a treadmill having not eaten all day will burn a small amount of fat as a fuel source, however the proportion of fat it uses will be severely diminished to there being a lack of glycogen in the muscles to be metabolised alongside the fat. You clearly want to be burning primarily fat remember! This means that you should have taken in some form of complex carbohydrates in the run up to your gym session.

Remember too that of this six hours glycogen supply, 25% of that is reserved for the brain and not the muscles, since the brain is only capable of using glucose from glycogen for energy. That's correct; your brain is incapable of using energy from fat or protein for fuel.

This really gives you 4.5 hours maximum of glycogen supply for your muscles. And this is if you're not being active. Ever wondered why you feel hungry after around 4 hours after your last meal?

However, in actual fact this will transpire to around 60 – 90 minutes of moderately hard activity at best!

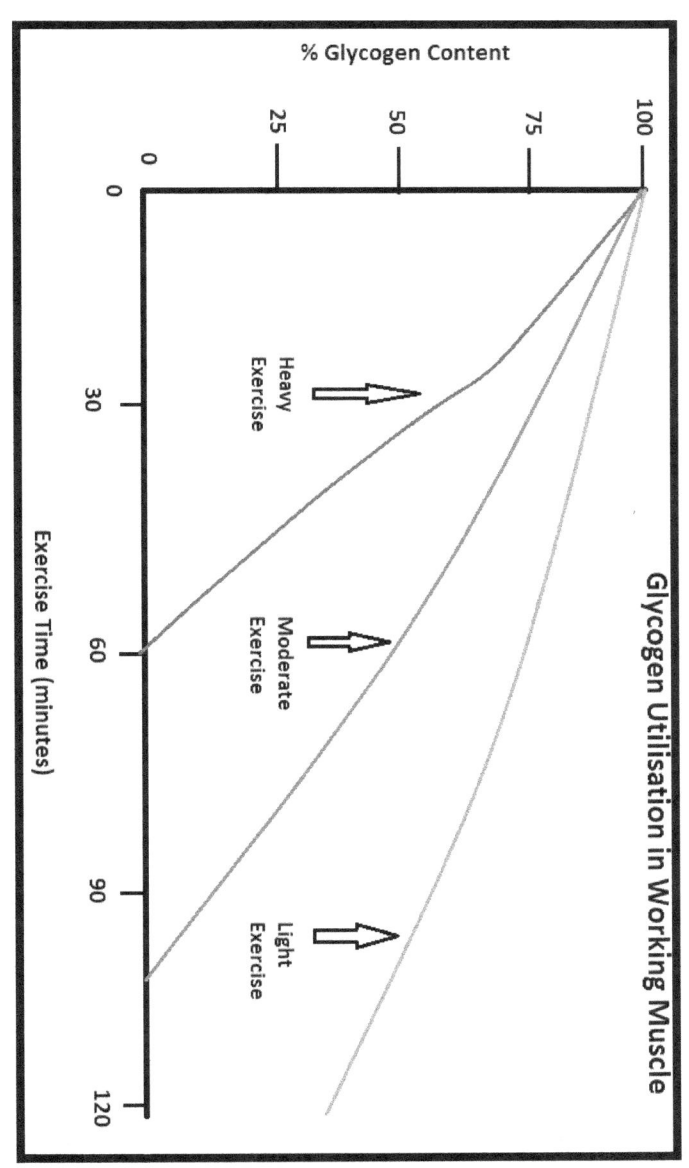

So what should we do?

Well clearly if we wait until we are hungry before we eat then we are already diminishing our ability to be burning fat, especially if we are planning some physical activity. Eating three or four large meals a day leaves us at risk of leaving that gap, especially if we are going for a workout. Not only that, but the body cannot cope with large amounts of food in one go, so if you wait until you're really hungry before eating you will most likely end up over consuming and end up with large fat storage as a result, not to mention a reduced workout performance due to being full.

By far the best thing to do would be to increase the amount of meals you have every day and decrease the quantity of food per meal.

It is far preferential for weight loss, as well as general good health to eat seven or eight smaller meals per day as opposed to two, three or four larger meals.

Ever wondered why you feel tired and sluggish after a large meal? It's because it takes a large amount of blood to digest large quantities of food and this is blood which is diverted away from your brain and your muscles, but is instead concentrating around your gut. In many countries, taking siestas has become part of the culture but this is just not very healthy. By eating smaller amounts more regularly you'll feel a lot better and more energetic as you go about your life.

In addition to feeling better, you'll be storing a lot less fat as well! Remember that excess glycogen will be converted to fat for later use. When you eat large meals there will be a lot of excess glycogen. By eating smaller yet more regular meals, your body will not be needing to convert this glycogen to fat, you'll have glycogen in your muscles to power your workout whenever you decide to take it, not to mention your daily activities and you'll feel more energetic too.

Triple whammy!

This is what I recommend to you...

I know that it takes discipline to stop eating when you're not full up, but this is what you're going to have to get used to doing! Try and spread your meals out throughout the day. Unfortunately, this may not be easy for many people depending on their jobs, but it's of vital importance that you try and make an effort; your health is after all at stake.

Of course, these smaller and more regular meals should be at least 60% complex carbohydrate based.

In fact simply by raising the amount of complex carbohydrates in your diet to 60%, assuming you are one of the majority who don't quite get that much and by spreading out your meals as suggested, you will almost certainly find that you'll be losing weight without even carrying out any exercise at all. This will be true even if you feel like you are actually eating a greater quantity of food. This is because as we know fat contains 9 calories to the gram whereas carbohydrates contain only 4. Also consider the increased TEF factor in carbohydrate when compared to fat.

If you're one of the one in three people who skip breakfast, I recommend you think again and try and make an effort. Porridge oats are one of the best sources of complex carbohydrates there is, they contain fibre also and so will fill you up.

If you take an early morning training session after having skipped breakfast, remember that you've already gone all night without eating as it is. This means it is too late for you unless you give yourself that early morning boost. Porridge is perfect for this! If not then you'll be having an extremely inefficient training session, burning minimal fat as fuel but instead using your body's lean muscle tissue instead. This is not what we're aiming for here.

I understand that it's difficult to exercise on a full stomach, but remember that I'm not asking you to exercise on a "full stomach" but instead a half full stomach which I would hope you'd be able to manage with ease. This will greatly boost your exercise performance, your mood, spare your protein supplies and lean muscle tissue and instead force your body to melt the fat from itself. Then don't forget that as soon as your training session is over, eat something else containing predominantly complex carbohydrates with a quantity of protein too.

Food High in Complex Carbohydrates

We've spoken about it, so now would be a fitting place to list foods high in complex carbs:

- Wholemeal/wholewheat bread
- Pitta
- Crackers
- Wholegrain Pasta
- Brown Rice
- Weetabix
- Porridge Oats
- Potatoes
- Broccoli
- Sweet corn
- Beans
- Tomatoes
- Sprouts
- Carrots
- Kidney Beans
- Lentils
- Bananas
- Nutrigrain Bars

Summary

- Fat cannot be metabolised on its own, but can only be metabolised in high proportions alongside carbohydrates.

- The exact proportion of fat metabolism depends on your activity levels.

- A greater proportion of fat to carbohydrate is used for energy the lower the activity levels, approaching an intensity of 60 - 65% maximal heart rate, when carbohydrate becomes the main fuel source.

- The more you train, the greater potential your body has for using fat as the primary fuel source.

- The exact proportion of fat metabolism depends also on the amount of glycogen in your muscle cells.

- When glycogen supply runs out, the level of fat metabolism decreases significantly and will instead use protein for fuel straight from your lean muscle tissue.

- This is bad because your muscles are used to actually metabolise fat in the first place. This is also bad because you're not burning as much fat as you could be doing if you're trying to lose weight.

- Your muscles can store only 6 hours maximum worth of glycogen at any one time, this is if you're being inactive.

- In reality 25% of this supply is reserved for your brain. This leaves about 4 hours of glycogen supply for inactive people.

- For the more active people, or for those with active jobs, glycogen stores can actually last for as short a time as 60 - 90 minutes.

- Always take in some form of complex carbohydrate in the time before your gym session. This will greatly raise the proportion of fat used as fuel.

Why Dieting Fails

If you've read the above few sections very carefully then you'll have a good idea already why dieting fails.

If you keep in mind that the whole point of dieting is not to "lose weight" but more specifically to lose *fat* then you should be able to hazard a good guess by now as to why bad dieting practices almost always fail. Let's take a look at the whole physiology and mind-set of the dieter a little more closely now.

Society puts incredible pressure on both men and women to be thin as thin is seen as the "ideal" way to be. Unfortunately the places (magazines, TV, newspapers etc) where these images of thin people being pushed as the desirable body shape are also often the same places where really bad advice to achieve such a figure is often dispensed and often by unqualified individuals.

These magazines will put images of ultra-thin models on the covers, not to mention on the inside, they will be dressed in all the latest designer clothes and then elsewhere in the magazine you'll no doubt read about the former obese lady who just lost eight stones in 3 months. You'll naturally feel under pressure to replicate this for yourself so that you could fit into the latest designer clothes.

As a personal trainer of many years, I know the most common question I'm asked is "How can I make my bottom/thighs/hips/belly smaller?"

It is often an uphill struggle to convince women who read bad advice in glossy magazines with their multi-million pound or dollar marketing budget that they are wrong and I am right and that they really should stop listening to their "dieting" advice.

Remember what I said about genetics earlier? Recent research has made some incredible findings into what determines how fat we will become and how easy or hard it will be to lose that fat. This research is very handy when it comes to developing fitness programmes for clients.

There are three main body shapes which fall into three categories. We all without exception are one of these body shapes although it's possible to be a mixture of two or even three, they are:

Ectomorphs – Tend to be taller with longer limbs compared to their bodies.

Mesomorphs – Have average proportioned limbs to their bodies and tend to be athletic.

Endomorphs – These are more rounded with shorter limbs compared to the rest of their bodies.

Unfortunately, at the time of writing this, there is absolutely nothing that we can do to alter our body shapes, short of employing a medieval torture/stretch rack.

With the bodies we are born with, we can make them look bigger or smaller, fitter or fatter, however it will absolutely always have the same proportions of limbs to body. Also, when we lose weight, our bodies will still have the same proportions, we won't look like anybody else, we'll just look like a smaller version of ourselves.

It may come as no surprise then that the amount of fat cells we have in our bodies, and where exactly these fat cells congregate is also determined by our genetics and our body types. Just look at where men and women differ in where they store fat; men tending to store it around their bellies and women tending to store it around their thighs. It is also known that different races of people store fat in different locations too. Of course also the different body types listed above will have a tendency to store fat in different locations and in different quantities. Fatter people don't necessarily have more fat cells than thinner people, it's more of a case of the existing fat cells that they have are more full of fat.

The resistance of these fat cells to losing the fat is also genetically determined. You may well be one of these people who have tried dieting in the past in an attempt to lose fat from a specific area, only to find that it drops off in other places but not where you wanted it to drop off from. This has the effect of making the target area look even bigger than before, especially in relation to the rest of you.

Recent research into obesity, its causes and effects have shown that the vast majority of people who try to diet, over many years actually end up within 1 or 2% of their starting weight, in addition to 1 or 2% of their body fat. All this despite much "advice" on dieting not to mention weight loss and exercise regimens from the poor people involved. All I can say is that it's a good thing you're reading this book, so you can avoid becoming one of these statistics.

So what are the mechanisms which control how fat we are? Well research suggests that we have a physiological mechanism living within our fat cells which in normal conditions will serve to keep our fat and body weight close to a genetic set point. This mechanism is easily able to cope with minor fluctuations which occur from day to day in our bodies or even with a weekend of binge drinking, cake eating or even starvation.

It is now known that our fat cells create a hormone called leptin. Leptin serves to speed up our metabolisms since it is triggered into synthesis when we eat. You know that feeling of being full? That is leptin telling your brain to stop eating! That is its other function in your body. It effectively acts as an appetite suppressant and an all-natural one too.

When your fat cells are as full up as genetics has deemed they should be, then you'll be producing leptin in the correct doses and your metabolism and appetite will be normal.

If the amount of fat in your fat cells increases to a slightly higher than normal level then the amount of leptin produced will increase which will increase your metabolic rate and decrease your appetite, quickly bringing everything back to normal and more acceptable levels again.

On the flip side, following a day of not eating very much at all, our fat cells will produce less leptin as the amount of fat in our fat cells decreases which will lead to a decrease in our metabolic rate, an increase in our appetite and once again everything will return to a normal level.

If we listen to this mechanism then it will work very well, causing us to only eat when we are hungry. However we all know that that is not easy! As I'm sure you're aware, we all have complete control over our eating habits and we can easily override these physiological signals. After all, we don't only eat because we are hungry, but for many other reasons also.

If we overeat for an extended time period then our fat cells will continually over synthesise leptin. Leptin remember serves to speed up our metabolism and decrease our appetite. If we ignore these leptin signals being sent to our brain then we will have to live with a new, larger body size.

This all means that in order for us to return back to our former, more desirable body weight and shape, we have to do more than simply eat less food, we must also:

- Take a look at our issues that made us eat for comfort and not for sustenance.
- Bring in healthy and realistic diet and lifestyle patterns that can last us for the rest of our lives.
- Learn not to ignore, but to listen to our body's natural signals.

With so much information being bombarded at you it is very easy to be influenced by negative or detrimental "dieting" advice, recommendations from people you know or "trusted" media sources about the latest wonder diet that works miracles. Ever heard of; Atkins, low carb diets, low GI diets, detox diets, liquid diets, water diets, high protein diets? I'm sure there are many more, but my time is limited! I mean who wouldn't be tempted to try the latest "diet" used by a Hollywood movie "star" who's lost 3 stones after giving birth. What you have to remember is that these people have a certain genetic makeup in the first place which is obviously a great advantage and the reason they are chosen to become stars in the first place, not to mention the best personal trainers in the world who get top dollar to make these "stars" look great for a multi-million dollar post natal photo shoot only weeks after g ving birth.

The truth is that nearly all diets are based on calorie restriction, no matter how glossy the magazine makes it look, or no matter which temporary Hollywood star is advocating it.

In order to lose weight calorie expenditure must be greater than calorie input!

The thing is that most diets advise quite extreme restriction in calories in order to guarantee short term "success!" I mean, if they didn't put on the front cover of the magazine that you're "guaranteed" to lose three stones in six weeks then you probably wouldn't spend your money on the magazine. It is in fact this "too much, too soon" approach that instead will guarantee for you long term fat loss failure.

*Now here is a good time to make the following point. You bought this book because of the title "Lose Weight Fast!"
But let me make clear that fast weight loss is never permanent weight loss and I would never compromise your health by giving you "fast" weight loss advice that was not healthy or indeed permanent. So we're going to have to agree to slow the speed down to a level that is "fastest" while still being healthy but more importantly your results will be permanent. Trust me, this really is the best way! Carry on reading and you'll discover exactly why I had to make that point.*

Let's take the following example; Sarah who is 30 years old. She is 5ft 5 inches tall and weighs 70Kg or 11 stones. Sarah would like to go on a diet to lose some weight. She has just read in a glossy magazine with a huge marketing budget that if she restricts her calorie intake to just 1000 kcal a day then she will lose 6-8 lbs in one week. What's more, she really trusts this "diet" because she saw the magazine advertised on TV between her favourite soap opera, so it must work!

Let's have a look at how many calories Sarah would need to take in in order to give her body its basic energy requirements.

Basal Metabolic Rate = 70 X 25 kcals = 1750 kcals per day. This goes on the premise that each Kg of body weight requires 25 Kcals of energy per day; this is if you're sedentary.

Let's assume that Sarah is not a sedentary female but is just fairly inactive so we'll add on an extra 20% to take into account her job and lifestyle.

This brings us to 2100 Kcals a day that she needs to take in.

Now this "diet" in her glossy magazine has recommended to her that she only takes in 1000 calories per day. This is less than half of what she actually needs in order to remain healthy. But just as importantly is that her intake is actually below her basal metabolic rate, the rate of intake which is needed to make her function. It is actually considerably lower than her BMR.

Sarah's body will perceive this as starvation!

Sarah's body now goes into survival mode!

Well not only is Sarah's body now in survival mode but she will be feeling hungry and miserable too.

Survival kicks in as a physiological response to a life threatening situation, which is designed to ensure, no matter what and at all costs the continuation of life, the survival of the organism. The body has no choice but to make several changes in order to ensure that all available energy is made to last longer in order to protect the vital organs such as the brain.

Remember from earlier that the brain can only use glucose straight from carbohydrate for energy. This comes from the liver. It does not have its own stores of glycogen like other organs and the muscles have.

All of this energy supply would actually be used up on the very first day of this restrictive calorie diet. All glycogen in the muscles and liver would be gone.

Let's assume that the total amount of glycogen in the body; muscle and liver amounts to a total of 250gms.

Glycogen is stored in the body in an extremely hydrated form. It requires 3gms of water for every 1gm of stored glycogen.

So what would Sarah's total weight loss be?

250gms glycogen + 3 X 250gms water = 1000gms = 1Kg / 2.2lbs.

But what exactly is the lost weight? It's all in the equation. Fat? A tiny bit! Carbs? Yes! Water? Yes!

But remember the body is in survival mode so because it is not getting the amount of calories it requires, it slows everything down:

BMR Drops!

This can be by as much as 20% and can occur in as quickly as 24 hours!

Remember that for fat loss programmes, we ideally want to be increasing our BMR, not decreasing it since BMR is essentially our free or weight loss for zero effort mechanism.

So instead of Sarah's daily calorie requirements being 25 kcal for every Kg of body weight, it has now reduced to 20 kcal for every Kg of body weight. This means that the calorie deficit created is now becoming lower and lower; Sarah literally needs less energy to survive because of this reduced BMR.

And this is after only one day of dieting!

On day two of Sarah's diet which she found in a glossy magazine, her energy needs will be reduced from day one due to the decrease in BMR. However, her energy needs are still above the supply that she is giving her body.

Most worryingly of all, her brain is lacking in glucose! This needs to be made urgently by the liver.

Glucose can quite easily be made by our bodies, but amino acids have to be broken down for this. Remember that there are no amino acids available due to the low calorie intake. So Sarah's body has to get them from somewhere else. So it will have to break down its own supply, straight from Sarah's lean muscle tissue. And here was me thinking the whole point of "dieting" was to lose fat.

Just like glycogen, muscle protein is also bound up with a lot of water. However, where with glycogen there is 3gms of water for every 1gm of glycogen, with protein there are 4gms of water for every 1gm of protein.

So for even a small amount of protein to be broken down to fuel Sarah's survival, say 100gms will mean a loss of lean muscle tissue to the sum of five times this amount; 500gms / 1lb in weight.

In only two days, Sarah has lost 2lbs of glycogen and 1lb in muscle. The sad thing too is that she'll have lost barely any fat into the bargain!

The body obviously doesn't like having to break down its muscle simply to sustain itself, so this is why it slows everything down, lowering your BMR, making you extremely tired and miserable. But make no mistake, until the body can get energy from somewhere, it will have no choice other than to catabolise your muscle to power itself. This muscle loss will be quite extensive, especially in the early weeks of a calorie restricted diet.

Without a doubt, weight loss in the first week of a calorie restricted diet will be primarily from your lean muscle tissue and its associated bound up water.

The sad thing is that your body has plenty of fat stores available which it could use, but it just can't. Here is why:

Fat is stored in our bodies in a very dehydrated form. Ever tried to mix water and fat or oil? They don't mix! In fact you would need to create a calorie deficit of 500 Kcals per day, every day to lose 1lb of fat a week which equates to 3500 Kcals.

Remember though that because the body cannot burn fat alone, a significant proportion of this deficit will need to come from carbohydrates.

Therefore, in order for Sarah to lose just one pound of fat a week, she would need to create a calorie deficit of roughly 750 Kcals a day. As we have already discussed, this 750 Kcal reduction in calories would put most people well below their BMR and therefore into starvation mode.

This would force the body to respond by:

- Inhibiting the activity of enzymes that release and burn fat.
- Increasing the activity of fat storage.

This is clearly not the goal of any decent weight loss regime.

As we know, the efficiency of fat burning decreases significantly when carbohydrate is not available.

So what will happen to poor Sarah next?

Well as the diet continues, weight loss will actually decrease! Why? To protect vital lean muscle tissue but also because of the physiological changes that will be occurring due to this starvation.

It may be that several weeks into her diet, no more weight loss will occur for Sarah. This is because she will have reached a plateau. The body has now learned to adapt to the new situation Sarah has placed herself under, although at a drastically decreased efficiency and she'll have all the associated health risks that go along with that.

You must understand also that throughout all this time, Sarah will have felt extremely tired and lethargic. She will have been miserable, she will have been less productive and quite possibly in pain. She will also have had to turn down any dinner invitations she may have received due to being on this new miracle "diet!"

But having now plateaued, what can she now do to "kick-start" the weight loss again? Well, because weight loss has slowed down almost to a stop on 1000 Kcals a day, perhaps she ought to go for 750 Kcals a day instead? Yes she could do this! Weight loss would indeed pick up again and she would lose even more of what she perceived to be "weight." Then after a short amount of time, perhaps a week or two, her body will then readapt to this new low level of calorie intake and then once again she will plateau.

I suppose then she could start taking in even less than 750, perhaps 500 kcals in order for the weight loss to continue.

However, when weight loss does eventually come to a stop, what most people tend to do is not reduce their calorie intake even further, what they do instead is to revert back to their old ways, resuming their normal calorific levels.

But wait - Sarah's body has become used to taking in 1000 kcals a day and now all of a sudden she is taking in 2100 kcals. Sarah's body perceives this as a "binge." A binge being many extra calories entering the body that the body just can't cope with, so what does the body do? It stores it as fat!

Not only that but because of the severe loss of lean muscle tissue that Sarah has undergone the previous month; she has now lost much of her fat burning potential. She will in effect be burning this new fat at a much slower rate than she would have if she never went on this miracle diet at all.

Sarah can now expect to put on even more weight, with much more ease than ever before. In addition, she'll find getting rid of her new fat even more difficult now.

In a year's time, Sarah is now heavier than she ever was, more miserable and with a lower self-esteem than ever before. So what does she do? She embarks on another diet! But this one must work great because she saw it in a glossy magazine and it's used by all the famous celebrities, some of whom have lost 3 stones in just a few weeks.

Ever heard the saying "I feel like I've been on a diet my whole life?"

This is the cycle that afflicts 95% of dieters throughout the world. This is the 95% that do not work! Luckily, because you're reading this book, you'll be one of the 5%!

Eating A Low Fat Diet

It should have been made clear by now that the aim is to reduce the amount of fat in our diets and doing so in a way that increases the amount of complex carbohydrates and fibre.

But buying products that are low in fat is becoming increasingly difficult; for example, many salads bought at the supermarket are actually extremely high in fat.

It is obvious that we need to be extremely vigilant when buying our food, we also need to know what to look out for when it comes to food labelling.

- Ensure you avoid all food containing trans fatty acids. They claim to be better than saturated fats but they are in fact much worse. They severely increase the bad cholesterol while decreasing the amount of good cholesterol in your body. Always check the label of any margarine, cakes or biscuits and avoid purchasing these items. It would be much better to buy butter rather than margarine containing trans fatty acids.
- Be wary of foods containing the word 'light' as under law, the manufacturer, depending in which country you live does not need to specify what they actually mean by this. Light could refer to a reduction in salt, sugar or alcohol. It could even mean that the product is lighter in colour.

- Likewise be wary of low fat claims as many countries do not have restrictions on claims they can put on their products labels.

It would be much better if you check the actual label of the products you're buying for actual fat content. This of course means having to do a little work when you go shopping, but within a couple of shopping trips, you'll be buying the same things and it will just be automatic for you.

Remember that your fat intake needs to be between 30 – 35% of your overall calorie intake. So any product that contains less than 30% fat should be considered low fat. By the way, many supermarket salads contain 40%+ fat, so you really do need to learn how to calculate fat content from reading the food labels as of course, they seldom help us out by placing the correct fat percentages on the label.

How to Calculate the Percent Calories of Fat Contained in a Product?

Let's take this 100g pack of Barbecue Beef flavoured Batchelors Super Noodles. I love these, they are very tasty:

Energy   2079kJ / 496kcal (per 100g)

Fat   22.2g

Carbohydrate   64.4g

Protein   9g

So we need to multiply the grams of fat by 9, since there are 9 kcals per gram of fat.

22.2 X 9 = 199.8kcals.

This brings us to a total of 199.8kcals from fat in a single pack of said Super Noodles.

Now we divide this number by the calories per serving/100 grams. Note that it needs to be per 100 grams which should be stated on the pack.

199.8 / 496kcal   =   0.40

Now simply multiply this number by 100.

0.40 X 100   =   40% fat content.

As you can see, we don't really need the carbohydrate or the protein content at all to work out fat percentage. I included those figures because it is easy to see how, despite the figure for carbohydrate being much larger in relation to fat, actually isn't that far off the same level; 52% considering you multiply the carbohydrate in grams by 4 and not 9.

Now let's take a look at a slightly easier yet not quite as accurate way of working this out on a carton of Longley Farm Natural Cottage Cheese.

Energy   434kJ / 104kcal (per 100g)

Fat	6.0g

Check that the product is below 3 grams of fat per 100kcals. If it is then it will certainly be below 30% fat since: 3 X 9 = 27 kcals! This is actually 27% of fat which is even better!

In the case of this cottage cheese, the actual fat content is 52%!

There is no need to try and eliminate fat from your diet altogether, in any case this will be impossible to achieve, but knowing this information, you'll at least be able to tell that the salad you've been buying for lunch a couple of times every week in the belief it was low fat is in fact extremely high in fat.

The truth is that in order to ensure a low fat meal, you'll probably have to prepare it yourself, knowing full well the fat content of the ingredients you're using.

There is no reason either that you have to substitute taste in order to have a low fat meal.

Follow these guidelines for helping you to modify your regular meals to low fat meals:

Quick and Easy Low Fat Meal Guidelines

- Substitute deep or shallow frying for baking, grilling, steaming and microwaving.
- Use oven chips/fries instead of deep frying chips/fries.
- If you need to use oil in your recipe, rather than pouring it on, try using a spray bottle and dispense it with that.
- If your recipe asks for whole eggs, use two egg whites for each single egg yolk.
- Use vegetable margarine instead of butter or lard.
- Substitute skimmed or low fat milk for whole milk, pasteurised or semi-skimmed. Trust me, you soon get used to skimmed milk and pretty soon you won't be able to tell the difference.
- Substitute cream for low fat yoghurt or fromage frais.
- Try 'Quark' cheese instead of cream cheese.
- Quit adding sugar to hot drinks.
- Always reduce the amount of sugar or fat the recipe asks for.
- Always reduce the amount of nuts too.
- If any recipe asks for mayonnaise, you should substitute this with low fat yoghurt or fromage frais. At the very least, use low fat mayonnaise.
- Substitute at least part of your flour for whole wheat flour.

- Reduce the amount of salt to half or less. Try to eliminate table salt entirely.
- Try and halve the amount of cheese you normally use.
- Substitute chips/fries for side salad.

Of course I'm all for enjoying life and a big part of this is eating out every now and then. Take some of the following into account:

- Burgers are lower in fat than fish/chicken sandwiches.
- Order burgers without cheese as this always greatly increases the fat content.
- Likewise, order your burgers without mayonnaise and other sauces.
- Avoid deep fried products at Chinese takeaways such as; spring rolls, fried noodles or anything with skin.
- When eating at Indian restaurants, bear in mind that many of the sauces contain cream. Avoid korma and other creamy sauces.
- If you go to McDonalds, substitute your Big Mac (47% fat) for a hamburger (32% fat).

Fast Weight Loss Diet – Summary

We have covered a lot of ground in this section when it comes to diet. If you've kept up and understood everything then congratulations, you'll just need to put everything into action now.

To make things easier for you, I have summarised the main points you need to remember below:

- To lose weight you need to expend more energy through metabolism, digestion, activity and exercise than you take in through food.
- The recommended daily calorific intake is 2500 for males and 1800 for females.
- You should never reduce your daily calorific intake by more than 10%!
- You need to reduce your fat intake to the recommended daily amounts of between 30 – 35% of your total calorie intake. This is because fat is more energy dense than both carbohydrates and protein combined. Due to the thermic effect of food, we also expend less fat energy through the natural digestion process.
- Fat is also the least satiating of all the three main nutrients, filling you up the least. This is another reason to lower your fat intake.
- Carbohydrate should account for around 60% of total calorie intake.

- Protein should be around 10 or no more than 15% of total calorie intake.
- Increase fibre content in your diet. Fibre contains zero calories and will fill you up.
- Reduce the amount of simple or sweet sugars/carbohydrates from your diet. An abundance of this will lead to excess fat storage.
- Your diet should be as high as possible (60%) in complex carbohydrates. Most of these foods also contain fibre which will help to fill you up. Eating an excess will therefore be difficult and the body uses up energy to convert excess in this form into fat.
- So increase consumption of the following: bread, pitta, crackers, pasta, rice, Weetabix, porridge oats, potatoes, broccoli, sweet corn, beans, tomatoes, sprouts, carrots, kidney beans, lentils, bananas – Particularly wholegrain versions of these foods where possible.
- Increase your water intake. A good quantity to begin with is 5 pints a day and increase to around 7 – 8 pints per day within a few weeks. Adopt the little and often strategy; taking in a sip every ten or so minutes. Always have water by your side and aim to never feel thirsty. This will serve to fill you up so you'll eat less at meal time. Your body will also use up energy to process the water.
- Cut out fizzy drinks entirely from your diet!

- If you drink tea or coffee then ensure you drink an extra quantity of water to make up for this.
- Stop adding sugar to hot drinks.
- The human body cannot utilise fat for energy alone in any great quantity. It must be used in conjunction with carbohydrates.
- This means it's of vital importance to give yourself a regular supply of complex carbohydrates.
- Instead of eating three of four large meals per day, you should now be aiming to eat seven, eight or nine + very small meals. This will ensure a constant supply of glycogen for energy which will heighten fat usage too. This will also ensure a minimum amount of fat storage due to over filling.
- Finally, having adequate glycogen supply in your muscles will ensure an increased level of fat utilisation all day long. No matter if you're at work, watching TV or exercising.
- It's very important to have taken in some form of complex carbohydrates in the 30 minutes prior to exercising. Porridge works very well for this.

Section 3

Metabolism Out

We have spoken at length about the energy you will be taking in, what you should be eating, when, how often and how much.

If you follow all the advice so far in this book then trust me, you will find your body composition improving without even having to do very much exercise at all. This is because diet and eating correctly is a huge part of transforming yourself.

I understand that incorporating everything I've told you to do so far will be a big change for many, but this really is the fastest way to successful weight loss while remaining healthy. There has not been one thing that I've asked you to do in this book that will jeopardise your health in any way whatsoever. On the contrary; by changing your habits to what I suggest, you'll find yourself with a new lease of life, abundant in energy to a level you never thought possible. What's more, all this will be permanent. That is the difference between my strategy and all the other "lose weight quick" schemes you will read in glossy magazines, you know the ones that tell you to eat 1000 calories per day.

The next part of this book will now concentrate on your metabolism, speeding it up through a range of methods. This is the next big part of the puzzle; expending energy, burning fat and building muscle tone in the process.

Daily Activities

Much of this chapter will be common sense advice. Admittedly many reading this book may have heard much of this before. I include this chapter to emphasise just how important it is to burn off your calories through your everyday chores, activities, work and general living.

Take another look at the Fundamentals of Weight Loss scale:

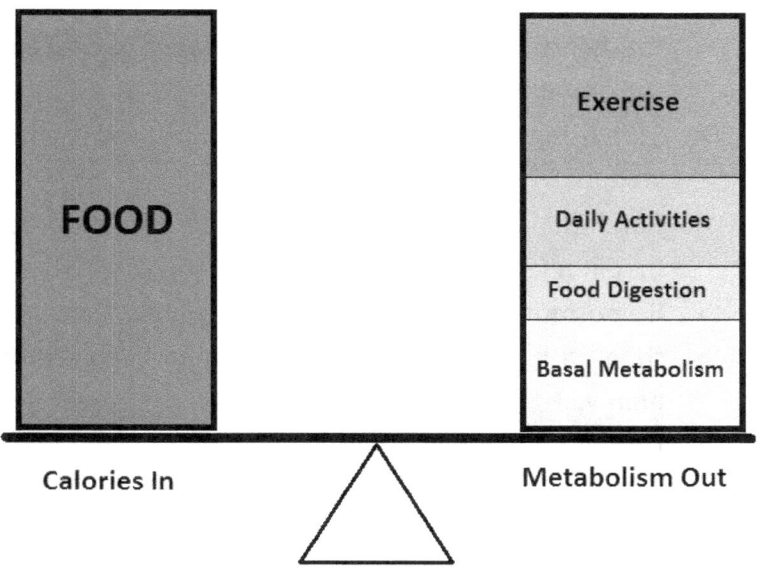

As you can see 'daily activities' is a big part of the equation. By increasing the amount of energy you expend simply by getting about and carrying out your business you can tip this scale further in the direction of weight loss.

But remember how modern society has made expending energy through every day methods increasingly difficult. We are going to have to buck the trend here and start making an effort. If you consider all the little things that are listed below, they will all soon add up to a massive amount that will make a great deal of difference to you.

To maximise weight loss through your everyday activities and everyday living, follow these tips:

- When walking anywhere, no matter how short a distance, simply speed up the pace a little to get the heart working that little bit harder, increasing the amount of calories used.
- Stop using elevators and escalators. Instead use the stairs.
- Purchase a bicycle and use that for short or medium length journeys instead of the car.
- If you must drive to work, or use public transport then park or get off the bus at an earlier position and walk the rest of the way.
- During your lunch break, don't stay at your desk but instead take a short walk. Just ten or fifteen minutes a day will make you more alert and the calories will add up over the course of the following months.
- If you're sat at a desk for long periods, take breaks every hour to walk around the office for a few minutes.

- For future family outings, why not make them physical? Long walks in the countryside or national park, skiing, paintballing, swimming etc.
- Isn't it annoying when going to the supermarket that you can never find a car park spot close to the entrance? Well simply park your car at the furthest point to the entrance and take a brisk walk there instead. Problem solved!
- When carrying out any household chores; vacuuming, washing the car, cleaning the bathroom etc, simply increase the pace to make it more of a workout.

Common Activities and their Intensity

In 2000, Ainsworth et al published their incredible work on the Compendium of Physical Activities. In this, they graded the level of physical exertion in a range of activities and occupations on a scale of <1 to 20. Where 1 is considered resting and every incremental whole number thereafter is considered a multiple of 1 in intensity. The lowest level of physical exertion was of course found to be sleeping which was graded at 0.9. The highest recorded level was 18 which was found to be running at 10.9 mph.

The compendium is an excellent way of finding out just how hard you're actually working when you carry out your household chores in relation to certain exercise activities and it does indeed make surprising and interesting reading.

For example, vigorous sexual activity unfortunately is classed only as a 1.5 on the scale. This destroys the myth that sex is a good workout.

There are many hundreds and thousands of activities included in the compendium, so I have singled out the most intensive as well as some of the most common everyday activities here along with their relative intensity.

1.5   Bathing

2.0   Showering

2.0   Dressing

2.0	Cooking
2.0	Making the bed
2.3	Ironing
2.3	Food shopping
2.3	Washing dishes
2.5	Watering plants
2.5	Playing piano
3.0	Playing guitar
3.3	Sweeping floors
3.5	Vacuuming
3.5	Mopping
3.8	Scrubbing floors
3.9	Washing car, windows
4.0	Playing drums
2.5 - 5.0	Playing with children
2.5 - 5.0	Playing with animals
5.0	Cleaning gutters
5.0	Painting walls
5.5	Mowing lawn

6.0   Moving furniture

7.5   Carrying groceries upstairs

9.0   Moving household items upstairs

Of course, simply by carrying out each of these chores with more gusto (where possible) you can increase the intensity significantly.

Low Intensity versus High Intensity

Now, I feel that I really need to further clarify myself in this very important section. Earlier in this book I said the following:

"As you can see, fat utilisation is higher at the lower intensities and declines as the activity becomes more intense. There is though a caveat to this rule that I will explain later on, why I still advocate for higher intensity activities for increased fat burning. You will find out why later on and it will change your entire mind set to exercise."

Yes it is true that the proportion of fat burned to carbohydrate is higher the lower the intensity of exercise. I made the above point however not to emphasise that you should be carrying out only low intensity activity to burn fat, but more to make the point that you really do need to have high glycogen concentrations in your blood and muscles to maximise fat burning. That is true no matter what the intensity of exercise may be.

But I want you to realise that when it comes to trying to burn off fat through cardiovascular exercise; it is always better to increase the intensity of the exercise, even if this means decreasing the overall duration.

Yes this will indeed burn off a greater proportion of carbohydrate when compared to fat. But I want you to consider the fact that by increasing your exercise intensity, you will be disproportionately increasing the number of total calories burned.

Yes, a lower percentage of these total calories will be fat calories, but from a far greater number. The result will be that in fact a higher number of fat calories will end up being metabolised in total.

30 mins - medium intensity running	30 mins - high intensity running
Total calories metabolised = 350	Total calories metabolised = 550
Fat / Carbohydrate = 50 / 50%	Fat / Carbohydrate = 40 / 60%
Total = 175 / 175	Total = 220 / 330

The above example is completely subjective and the total calories and exact proportions of fat to carbohydrate metabolised will be dependent on many factors. But I hope I've made my point that you will burn more fat calories as well as total energy by increasing the intensity of exercise.

But this isn't the only mechanism by which you'll be increasing the amount of fat you'll be burning both at the time of exercise and in the future by increasing the exercise intensity.

The law of evolution states that for organisms to change and evolve, the organism must first be placed under stress. For the greatest amount of change to take place, there must be a greater amount of stress.

This stress is high intensity work!

I'm afraid that low or even moderate intensity cardiovascular work just doesn't place the human body under anywhere near enough stress for it to make the degree of change that you would most desire and in a time frame that matches the title of this book. But by working at high intensities and by feeling that painful lactic acid building up and burning you and hurting you, then this will force your body to change at an extremely elevated rate.

There are in fact three mechanisms by which high intensity work will increase the rate of fat loss over low intensity work. The first I have explained above. Now let's talk about the other two.

To better explain these mechanisms I'm going to lift a couple of chapters from my best-selling book *HIIT – High Intensity Interval Training Explained.* There is no greater method in existence for obliterating the fat from your body. How much do I believe in the power of HIIT? Well I wrote an entire book just on that subject!

As I will of course be recommending HIIT to you for your weight loss regime, I will explain it to you in this book. But for now, let's learn a little about its fat burning power. Here is an excerpt from *HIIT.*

Increase in Mitochondria

The first of those mechanisms is the increase in the number of and the size of the existing mitochondria within the muscle cells.

Mitochondria are known as the cells "power houses" as this is where glycogen is oxidised and energy is created. When we exercise, over time the increase in mitochondria and their efficiency enhances the body's ability to burn fat for us.

So how does this increased capacity compare between HIIT and CT (continuous training or medium intensity training)? Let's have a look at a study:

At the University of Guelph, Ontario in 2008 the study was intended to observe HIIT and its ability to improve the body's fat and carbohydrate metabolic capacities in untrained individuals.

The subjects took part in 10 x 4 minute bouts of high intensity cycling separated by 2 minute recovery periods. Exercise sessions took place 3 days a week for a duration of 6 weeks.

At the end of the study, a resting muscle biopsy was taken and there were found to be increases in citrate synthase (26%), a mitochondrial enzyme and 2 different fat transport proteins (14% & 30%). It was found that while cycling at a steady pace of 60% of their maximal heart rate potential, there was a marked increase in fat and carbohydrate oxidation capabilities.

Unfortunately, one limitation of the study was that it did not compare HIIT subjects with CT subjects which would have been interesting.

Just to clarify also, the study showed that the marked increase in fat and carbohydrate oxidation capabilities was for CT workouts *after* the HIIT sessions. This shows that after performing HIIT for a period of time and then returning to CT, your body has become more efficient at burning fat.

In another study at the same university in 2006, 8 women took part in 10 x 4 bouts of high intensity cycling with two minute recovery periods.

The subjects took part in 7 exercise sessions over a two week period.

At the end of the study, fat oxidation capabilities had increased by 36%.

Yet again unfortunately, there was no CT group to compare results to. You think they would have learned their lessons at this university but the good thing that came out of the study was that you can see incredible increases in fat burning potential after only 7 exercise sessions. This is the power of HIIT.

However I will now bring your attention to another study that took place at McMaster University in Ontario in 2006. I'm assuming there must be some kind of rivalry between the Ontario institutions to become the authority in HIIT research.

Anyway, 16 men were randomly assigned to either a HIIT group or a CT group. Each group performed 6 training sessions over 14 days on a bike. The HIIT group took part in 4 – 6 x 30 second all out bouts of exercise with 4 minute recovery periods between. The CT group took part in 90 – 120 minute bouts at around 65% of their maximal heart rate.

The muscle biopsy samples taken before and after the study showed that there were similar increases in fat and carbohydrate oxidative capacity in both groups.

But yet again, do you notice anything strange with the study above?

Take another look at the overall exercise durations for both groups because the differences here are massive indeed. The HIIT groups exercise sessions lasted for an average of 22.5 minutes compared to the CT group which lasted for 105 minutes. Over the duration of the study this works out at 2 hours 15 minutes (HIIT) and 10 hours 30 minutes (CT).

There you have it - With only a fraction of exercise duration, HIIT is comparable to CT when it comes to increasing muscle fat and carbohydrate oxidative capacity.

Excess Post-Exercise Oxygen Consumption (EPOC)

The final mechanism I referred to is termed *oxygen debt* or *excess post exercise oxygen consumption* (EPOC). If you read a lot on the subject of health and fitness then you may commonly hear EPOC described as the *after burn effect*.

When you exercise on full burners as you would with a HIIT session, the aerobic system alone cannot possibly supply you with enough energy to fuel the activity. Although it will do its best and give you all it has, the anaerobic system will have no choice but to come into play to provide extra energy assistance. This point typically comes in at between 65 – 85% of your maximal heart rate, as we'll discuss in the next section.

I will explain the principle of EPOC with the help of an example. Imagine you were going for a swim from one side of a lake to the other. You knew it would take an hour to complete this swim so naturally, you decide to pace yourself. Even if it was your goal to reach the other side of the lake in as fast a time as possible, you would still pace yourself so you wouldn't run out of energy too soon. But what if a shark suddenly appeared and started to swim towards you? Luckily you see a large rock directly in front, about a minutes swim away; so you turn on the full throttle and give it everything you have to reach the rock in order to save your life.

Now, would you say you would be breathing harder after reaching the rock or after reaching the other side of the lake? Of course the answer is that you'd be breathing harder after reaching the rock. This is because turning on full burners has placed immediate and great stress on your aerobic metabolism; this is partly why you're breathing so hard.

A very basic evolutionary and physiological principle is that your body adapts to stress. So if you escape from sharks on a regular basis, or better yet, mimic the shark part in a more controlled environment such as a swimming pool then your body is going to change for the better.

Another reason why you are now breathing harder after reaching the rock than when you reach the end of the lake is because you are now requiring additional oxygen to replenish significant energy stores that were used in haste via non-oxidative metabolic pathways (see Energy Systems below) in order to save you from the shark.

Now this part is very important; you will now need to deal with the incredibly large amounts of lactic acid that have built up in your muscles during the swim as a result of turning on the full throttle. The build-up of lactic acid has had nothing to do with the duration of the swim at all, but is there solely due to the high intensity of the swimming, having escaped from the shark.

This elevated level of oxygen consumption, which will last for several hours, will continue to have a training effect on the body. This is what is meant by the term EPOC or the *after burn effect*. You have finished training, yet you are still burning fuel or calories at an elevated rate due to the high intensity of the activity.

Let me reiterate that there is no EPOC from CT (Continuous Training/exercise at lower intensities) because the activity is just not intensive enough. EPOC is only gained after high intensity activity. How long will EPOC last for? That all depends on exactly how intense the activity was. The more intense the activity – The greater the EPOC. Naturally, the effect of EPOC is at its maximum during the first few hours post exercise when the body has the greatest need to recover. The effect of EPOC then gradually diminishes over and up to the next 48 hours – The harder the intensity of the prior activity, the longer EPOC lasts.

Metabolic Rate

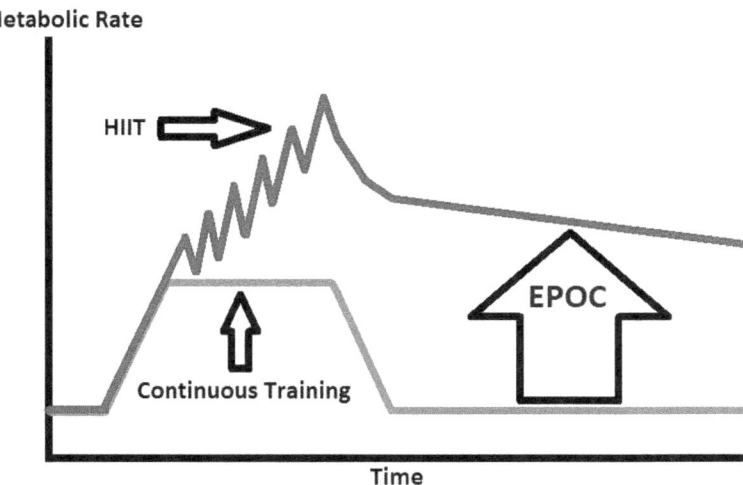

Are you now imagining the physiological benefits that are possible by engaging in regular and sustained HIIT? The potential is massive.

So why else are there such incredible differences in improvements between HIIT and CT?

Well this has to do with the body's energy systems. There are three energy systems in total; the ATP system, the glycogen or lactic acid system, finally there is the aerobic system.

Energy Systems

Each system uses fat and carbohydrate for fuel in different frequencies. Each system is used in different proportions depending on the exercise intensity. They are working all the time in the background and slide in and out of action depending on what we're doing.

The ATP system is used for high intensity work such as sprinting and lasts usually for 10 seconds or less before becoming depleted. The term ATP refers to *adenosine triphosphate* which is in rare supply in the body, but don't worry, once it runs out the body can quickly make it again, luckily for those who do HIIT regularly.

The glycogen/lactic acid system lasts for a bit longer, usually for between 30 seconds to up to 3 minutes and beyond depending on your fitness. Glycogen is the body's supply of fuel which it uses for everything; it tends to be made available to order.

The aerobic system is the system we use the vast majority of the time; when we're eating, sleeping, watching TV or performing very light to moderate exercise.

When we perform CT for long periods, we are only in effect using the one energy system; the aerobic system. It's only when we cross the 65 – 85+% of our maximal heart rate threshold (depending on how fit you are) does the glycogen system come into play. This is where we are in effect utilizing energy on two levels. This is the spot we must aim to hit (or even higher), albeit for only a short duration when partaking in HIIT. In fact in HIIT we should aim to go for 100% of our maximal heart rate in order to train our ATP system also. This way we're utilizing energy on three levels, not two and not one.

Unlike CT, HIIT gives a workout to all three energy systems and not just the aerobic system. This gives us an all-round better workout and has many physical benefits for us that a less interesting CT session can't touch.

By participating in HIIT, you receive a large increase in post exercise fat burning over and above what CT can do. You should think of this as free training time because you have ended your workout session, but your body is still burning fat at an elevated rate.

To clarify this point a little more, I'll mention a study that showed that 24 hours after a HIIT session, HIIT subjects were still burning calories at an elevated rate, whereas the CT subjects were not. Over the 24 hour period that followed HIIT sessions, this equated to an extra 100 calories burned over the CT group. This is quite significant and why HIIT participants can burn more energy and lose more fat by carrying out a lot less work than CT participants.

To really hammer home the fact that you continue to burn fat at an extremely elevated rate following HIIT workouts, I will mention another study that took place at Laval University in Quebec in 1994. The study was designed to discover the outcome of CT and HIIT on body fatness and muscle metabolism.

32 men and women were assigned randomly to a CT group or a HIIT group. The CT group took part in a 20 week programme whereas the HIIT group took part in a 15 week programme. By the end of the protocol, the mean estimated energy cost of the CT group was 120.4 MJ and the mean estimated energy cost of the HIIT group was 57.9 MJ.

Now consider that these figures represent the energy cost from the exercise activities only and not with the inclusion of EPOC. Consider also that the CT group's exercise programme lasted for a full 5 weeks longer than that of the HIIT group. This isn't how I would have designed the study, but let's run with this.

At the end of the study, body fat skin fold measurements were taken and the HIIT group were found to have undergone a reduction in body fat a full nine times greater than that of the CT group.

Read that again.

Nine times greater!

All this despite the amount of energy actually used during the exercise activities were more than two times greater in the CT group over the HIIT group.

Clearly the only way this can be explained is that there are energy sapping physiological changes taking place only following exercise that produces high quantities of lactic acid (HIIT). It further goes to prove that it's not about the duration of exercise, but the intensity.

I'm sure you've heard of the old saying "no pain – no gain" which was coined by Benjamin Franklin.

It appears it really is the truth.

End ^^^

If you would like to read the rest of the book, as well as the studies I have referenced, then I really do recommend my book *HIIT – High Intensity Interval Training Explained*. I will give the full description at the end of this book. Although I must emphasise that you don't need to purchase the book because of course, I fully intend on explaining the HIIT concepts in this book.

It really is the truth - HIIT is by far the most superior training method you can possibly partake in if your goal is weight or more specifically fat loss.

HIIT sessions generally take up much less time than normal run of the mill cardio sessions where you're running on a boring treadmill for 45+ minutes at a time.

It's been proven that you continue to burn fat at an elevated rate for many hours following a HIIT session. So even if you do have an hour long cardio session and let's say for instance that you burned off 500 – 600 fat calories, and the same again in carbohydrate calories; a simple HIIT session lasting between 20 – 30 minutes will do all that and more.

High Intensity Interval Training (HIIT)

This is the big one - This is the greatest tool in the weight loss arsenal!

It's a crime that HIIT is not more renown, but rest assured, more and more people are beginning to train via HIIT methods every day. The truth is slowly emerging as to the power of HIIT.

The problem is that there has been many years of fitness industry dogma which has named "cardiovascular training" or "aerobic training" as the only mode for weight loss. After all, it's in the name isn't it.

Yet the vast majority of professional athletes use HIIT all the time to train with.

In my book *HIIT*, I demonstrate that HIIT is superior to continuous training (CT) in every single fitness related category. If you can think of any aim or fitness related goal, then HIIT is the superior training method. Consider the following common fitness related goals:

- Athletic performance – HIIT gives better tolerance to lactic acid which is a hindrance to improved athletic performance. Any athlete who can better tolerate lactate build ups will have an advantage over his or her opponents.
- Weight loss – I even showed that HIIT was superior to CT for weight loss even within the exercise

session itself and not taking into account EPOC which helps to burn fat after the exercise session and increase in mitochondria (see weight loss potential below).

- Weight loss potential – Through EPOC and increased oxidation rates. This has been explained in detail above and is the true reason why with HIIT you continue to burn fat at extremely elevated rates for hours following the HIIT session.
- Improved anaerobic threshold – Which increases ones tolerance to high intensity work. Having a higher tolerance to high intensity work will be better for athletic performance (see above) and also for everybody else. This is true especially if you're particularly untrained as carrying out everyday tasks and chores can be exhausting.
- Increased VO2 Max – This is the best method of testing actual fitness. VO2 max refers to the body's ability to transport oxygen to the working muscles, which in turn become better at utilising the oxygen. This can further increase fat loss.
- Endorphin levels – The natural feel good chemical. You create much higher levels of the chemical beta-endorphin with HIIT over CT which is a natural response to pain but as a side effect makes you feel euphoric.
- Motivation – Because it's more fun and interesting.

I also proved that all these goals could be achieved in less than half the time of a CT session. Since it is "lack of time" which is cited as the number 1 reason for none compliance to exercise programmes, this is a very important factor.

Why does HIIT work so well?

I've already told you the answer. It is very intense! It produces a lot of lactic acid and your body needs to adapt rapidly to that stimulus.

Yet HIIT is still manageable even by the most unfit individuals due to the rest intervals it involves. In *HIIT* I referenced studies where ten year old children were used as the test subjects, highly obese and untrained individuals, all the way up to elderly triple heart bypass patients.

Everybody can do HIIT.

Let's talk about the specifics now.

How To Do HIIT

HIIT involves very short high intensity bouts of exercise immediately followed by low intensity rest periods.

For example, you could sprint or jog at a very fast pace. When you reach a point where you feel you can't carry on, even if this is after only ten seconds, then you would slow down to a slow jog or even a walk.

This walk, termed a rest period, is used for your body to disperse of the lactic acid and for you to recover in order to prepare for your next high intensity period, which should be coming up.

There are no hard rules as to how long each of your high intensity periods should be. Your lactic acid build up will dictate this to you. Likewise, there are no rules to the length of your recovery period. You should set off again when you feel suitably recovered.

There are no hard rules as to the quantity of high intensity periods (and by default recovery periods) but in general anywhere between six and ten is normal. You can take anywhere between 20 – 40 minutes to achieve these intervals. This time does not include your warm up and cool down.

You can set your high intensity and recovery periods due to how you feel in the moment. Or you can use physical markers such as lamp posts, street signs or trees as your signal to change intensity.

Important: The key ingredient to HIIT is that you must work as hard as you possibly can, for as long as possible. In the context of running, we're talking about sprinting for as long as you're capable which will be between ten and twenty seconds for the vast majority of people.

We are trying to create a painful lactic acid build up to give your body a damn good reason to change for the better.

The variables you can manipulate in HIIT are as follows:

- Duration (time or distance) of high intensity interval.
- Intensity (speed, resistance) of high intensity interval.
- Duration of recovery interval.
- Intensity of recovery interval.
- Number of repetitions of both high intensity interval and recovery interval.
- Mode of HIIT: Running, cycling, swimming, rowing etc.

Some people reading this may think to themselves that they can't sprint or cycle very fast so they will not be able to do HIIT. Well this misses the point. It is not the relative speed that matters, as this will be different for everybody who takes part. It is the intensity that matters!

Some people will be working at an all-out 100% maximal intensity simply by going for a brisk jog, whereas for others, a sprint will be necessary. The fact is that both individuals would experience a similar training effect since the only factor that matters, once again, is intensity and not speed. Over the years, I have found this point to be consistently misunderstood with my clients.

When partaking in HIIT you will of course gain rapid improvements - It is important that in order to keep gaining these improvements that you keep your HIIT sessions intensive by carrying out regular modifications. All you need to do is keep on increasing your intensity as you become fitter and more accustomed to HIIT. You can increase your intensity in a manner of ways such as by ensuring you're working to your full capacities, by decreasing the duration of recovery intervals, by increasing the quantity of intervals and even by changing training mode, say from running/sprinting to cycling or swimming.

HIIT Frequency

Apart from all the incredible improvements in health you can attain from HIIT, the other great thing about it is that you can do so without having to put in all that many sessions. You don't even need to put in that much time during each HIIT session either.

So what is the recommendation when it comes to HIIT frequency?

Well, because of the high intensive nature of HIIT and the body's need for recovery, I would recommend you partake no more often than every other day. In fact, every other day is the absolute most you should be doing it.

Like strength training a specific muscle in the gym, you would not work that same muscle on two consecutive days. Why? Because it needs sufficient time to rest and recover. It is exactly the same with HIIT. Your body needs rest.

Yes, three sessions per week is ideal for you if your goal is weight loss.

So how about the length of your actual HIIT sessions?

As you can see from the studies I've referenced, you can achieve all the wonderful benefits from a maximum of 30 minutes per session. I would therefore recommend that you go with 30 minutes. Certainly as you go above 30 minutes the law of diminishing returns seems to come into play. There is also the issue of the muscle's glycogen stores, which when working out at high intensities will deplete quickly. Once that happens then performance typically drops, muscle wastage begins and fat burning plummets – Not what we're trying to achieve with HIIT or for a weight loss regime.

A typical 30 minutes of HIIT should not include your warm up, cool down and stretches; you should consider those separate. We need 30 minutes of hard action here.

The number of intervals you're able to cram into a 30 minute HIIT workout will differ for everybody and will depend on many variables such as what your chosen activity is (running, cycling, rowing etc), whether you're in or outdoors, present state, HIIT experience and present fitness.

What is clear is that as you become more experienced and as your fitness improves, you should aim to decrease the duration of your recovery periods in order to cram one, two, three or even more high intensity intervals into a single workout. There's no need to increase the duration of a single HIIT session in order to squeeze in a few extra intervals. But you can certainly cram more high intensity intervals into a single 30 minute HIIT session.

Remember; quality, not quantity!

HIIT Modes

Now we're getting more into the practical side of things, we'll now take a look at some of the many possible HIIT modes.

The "best" training method will be completely down to the person involved. In reality, the HIIT training fundamentals can be used on nearly anything you can put 100% effort into; running, cycling, rowing, climbing the stairs or digging a giant hole in the sand.

I encourage everybody reading this book to try a number of different HIIT modes so you can find the modes which are dear to your heart. I recognise that most people, myself included will settle primarily on one single HIIT mode. However, as I'll explain in the summary section, there are extra benefits that can be attained simply by mixing up your training sessions. So please read through the following modes with an open mind and with a view to giving a few of them a fair go, even if you've never tried them before.

The training modes we're going to cover are as follows:

- Walking
- Running
- Cycling
- Rowing
- Skipping
- Stair Climbing

- Stepping
- Swimming
- Boxing
- Kettlebells
- Bodyweight Circuits

Walking

There'll be those who believe that HIIT can't be carried out while walking. To those people I would ask them if they've never walked up a large hill or a mountain with a heavy backpack.

Yes – HIIT can indeed be carried out walking and could in fact be the ideal starting point for the deconditioned individual, senior citizens or for those carrying injuries which are preventing them from running.

It is my belief that walking can be made intense enough for most people to achieve a HIIT training effect. But it should be made clear that when the individual is able to do so, then running should be made the primary focus.

While you'll see below that I don't really agree with HIIT running on a treadmill, with walking, using a treadmill will almost always be a necessity for HIIT. Most people will not be lucky enough to live next to a large hill or a mountain and so simulating these conditions using a treadmill will be essential. In order to achieve the required intensities while walking then for all but the most unconditioned individual - this will require a steep gradient.

Choose a brisk pace that will be a challenge and simply alter the gradients as necessary when entering your high intensity periods. Experimentation with making subsequent training sessions progressively more intense can be achieved by the use of ankle weights, weighted vests or by adding food cans or water bottles to backpacks. Of course, the speed of the treadmill can be altered too.

I must emphasise that if you feel unable to achieve the required high intensities when walking then you must consider some of the other training modes below.

Running

Running is the most popular mode for HIIT. It requires no equipment, no gym pass and unless you have an injury then everybody can do it, no excuses.

With running, you can change your speeds rapidly and easily, which is obviously beneficial for HIIT. It's also easy to set markers for yourself by using trees, lamp posts or any other landmark as signals to change speed.

While yes, you can do HIIT on a treadmill and many may prefer to do so, I personally have found changing the speed on most treadmills to be slow, inconvenient and perhaps a little dangerous. As you may know, there's a time lag when changing settings on many treadmills. If for example you've carried out a 10 – 20 second sprint, then you'll most likely really need to slow down quickly since spending any more time at a full sprint is extremely difficult even for the most trained of sprinters and you really don't want to be at the mercy of the treadmill when it comes to slowing down. In addition - stretching out your arms in order to change speed, while sprinting at full speed is more than a little risky. Of course there are many treadmills that enable you to pre-program your intervals which would eliminate the need to reach forward to change speeds. However, consider the possibility that you overestimate your sprinting capabilities and have to wait an extra 5 – 10 seconds at a high speed before the machine will automatically return to something more manageable. A lot to think about perhaps – But you can see why I much prefer pounding the grass outside instead.

You could get round this whole dilemma by maintaining a moderate speed on the treadmill and by using gradients. You can quite easily reach 100% of your maximal heart rate by maintaining a quick jogging pace or even a fast walk on a steep slope. So if your heart is set on using a treadmill then perhaps using a gradient will be the best compromise. Please make sure that you alter the gradient before the speed otherwise you may end up being surprised at just how hard it is to sprint up a steep gradient.

However, none of this compares to HIIT and sprinting outdoors where you can use real hills for your gradients and not be held back by having to fiddle with buttons when in full sprint mode.

Feel free to disagree with me when it comes to treadmill sprinting. I've had clients who've had no problems. But I wouldn't be doing my job if I didn't at least mention the above.

For those who decide to opt for the great outdoors, and I hope it's the vast majority, there are many things you can do to make your runs more interesting while at the same time adding extra elements of difficulty in order to ensure you're working at that magic 100%. Above all, gradients should be used as often as possible. Find a hill and use it. There are few more efficient ways of generating the required intensity than hill sprints. Likewise, sprinting through forests or along the beach will be more intense than sprinting on concrete. Packing a backpack with water bottles or food cans can work well too. They tend to roll and jump around the place, so be sure to pack towels or clothes in there to absorb the movement. Ankle weights can work in a similar fashion to a stuffed backpack.

I have one friend who built a customised sled that attached by rope to a weight lifting belt around his waist. He began by pulling along a 10kg weight in the sled. The weights then progressed to 20, 30 then 40kgs. After that he started at 10kg again, but this time he would pull the sled up a hill.

It typically takes him around 20 seconds to complete the run to the top of his hill. By that time he's long finished sprinting and has continued with a jog as fast as he can manage. When he reaches the top, he takes a leisurely walk back to the bottom, sometimes in an arc to give himself more recovery time. When he reaches the bottom, he begins again.

The moral is – You can always make your runs more interesting and more intense.

Cycling

Cycling is also a popular method for HIIT. In fact by cycling outside, you will often be performing interval training to a certain extent without even knowing it. This is because of the natural hills and troughs on any cycle route. Who pedals when going downhill anyway? Instead we tend to enjoy the thrill which would encompass a recovery period to my mind.

You can take this further by using your high intensity intervals to cycle harder or perhaps on a higher gear before changing to an easier gear and taking things easy for your recovery period. You should definitely utilise downhill slopes to recover.

Cycling on a stationary bike in a gym will be far preferential to using a treadmill in my opinion. Changing intensities is simple on a stationary bike; increasing speed on a high setting will be perfect for high intensity intervals, while taking things easy on a low setting will be ideal for recovery periods.

HIIT while cycling is great and you should definitely mix it in if you would normally prefer to run. Cycling is an ideal mode for the HIIT principles.

You can also take a spinning class. For those who don't know, spinning is an indoor group cycling session and most gyms these days will have classes running. Depending on the instructor involved, you will be taken through your paces at a range of intensities and speeds for around 45 minutes. Be warned; spinning is tough. It is also a lot of fun. You are in charge of setting your own intensities so you will be fully able to cycle at an intensity and speed that will succeed in giving you your lactic acid fix. Check the length of your spinning class. 45 minutes is a long time if you're going to be incorporating a HIIT workout into it. You should consider using the first half of such a session as a "warm up" by using a lower resistance on the bike. Then after the halfway point, crank up that resistance and go for it.

Rowing

In the vast majority of cases, rowing will be performed stationary unless you're lucky enough to live near a lake. Either you love rowing or you hate it and when it comes to HIIT, this is even more so. However, rowing will be another great mode to add to your HIIT inventory so I urge you to at least try it out.

Unlike with cycling, rowing utilises the whole body and so reaching those high intensities can be carried out with ease. Most people will agree that rowing can be incredibly intense, which is what we desire for HIIT.

Most rowing machines have a lever in order to alter stroke resistance. But the best way of increasing intensity is by increasing your stroke rate – effectively rowing faster. Between these two variables, you can make the intensities higher or lower as necessary.

For rowing, due to the position of the back, I must emphasise the use of correct technique and so I would recommend, if you've never used a rower before to speak to an instructor and learn correct form. You'll be pulling back on those handles with full force, straightening the knees at high speed. I must also emphasise that you should never lock out your knees on full extension otherwise this could cause problems down the line. Please have a trained instructor show you correct rowing posture and take you through your first attempt. It too often shocks me, watching people on rowing machines with appalling technique and posture.

However, if you have good fundamentals on this piece of equipment then you'll be able to achieve an incredible HIIT workout.

Skipping

Skipping is so simple. Anybody can skip or else learning can be done in no time at all. It's fun and it's free. Alternating your intensities is also a piece of cake.

I've had debates with other HIIT advocates as to which is the better mode for HIIT; running or skipping. I was on the side of running but it was a tough debate. Skipping certainly has its fans and extreme advocates. In fact, in the interest of changing things up, you should incorporate skipping into your workout every once in a while. Why not?

If you've never skipped before, or struggle with the technique, then keep everything slow until you become used to the mechanics. Keep the weight on your toes, try to be nice and light and make tiny jumps from the floor so you're not wasting any energy. There's no need to jump high when skipping.

I like to make use of a timer that beeps when it's time to change intensity. Others may wish to use an app on their phone. Otherwise you can simply position yourself facing a clock. Sometimes I will change the intensities depending on how I feel in the moment.

Obviously, to make skipping more intense, all you need to do is speed up. Then slow down to bring your heart rate back down again.

Stair Climbing

This is ideal for those who are pressed for time. Most of us have to climb a large flight of stairs during our working week at the office or even returning home to our apartments. If you can't fit in your HIIT sessions during the week, then sprinting up your flight of stairs will be the best compromise under the circumstances. At least you'll have no excuses for not taking some form of HIIT during the week.

Though using a long flight of stairs as your dedicated HIIT mode will of course work extremely well. There are few things more tiring than running up the stairs which makes this perfect for HIIT. When you get to the top, walk down again and repeat. Do this for a total of twenty minutes. If you would like to make this even more intense, although it's intense enough already, then you can employ the use of weights to hold while running or better yet you can purchase a weighted vest or fill a backpack with food cans or bottles of water.

I strongly hope you'll give stair climbing a try. It is after all about variety and experimenting with different modes to find which you enjoy the most and find more beneficial.

Stepping

Stepping is one of the more advanced methods which will not be ideal for everyone. Why? Because this exercise is extremely intense and vigorous, especially during high intensity periods.

By stepping, I'm not talking about the stepping machines you'll find in the cardio section at the gym, although they too can be used for HIIT. I'm talking about using an actual step.

Upright stepping involves the pattern of: One foot up, two feet up, one foot down, two feet down – Then repeat in rhythmical fashion for the desired training effect.

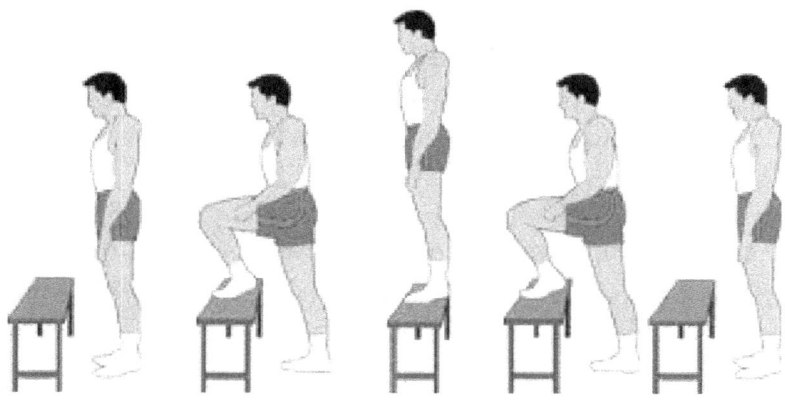

For the high intensity periods you will have a number of options in order to ramp up the heart rate. Most commonly, you can simply speed up the motion of the exercise. Another thing you could do is have a high step for the high intensity intervals and a low step for the recovery periods. You also have the option of using weights or a back pack filled with food cans or bottles of water. Why not use a combination of all these to truly make this an advanced mode of training?

Another advantage of stepping is that it can be carried out literally anywhere; the local park, in the home, hotel room and of course at the gym where setting up stepping boxes of various heights will be easy.

So why is this training mode so advanced when all that's involved is stepping?

Have you ever heard of *delayed onset muscle soreness* (DOMS)? DOMS is what happens following activity with prolonged eccentric movements. The term *eccentric* refers to controlled lowering movements. We perform controlled lowering movements when we put down heavy objects, run downhill or step.

Eccentric exercises cause DOMS, which is effectively a more painful fatigue which manifests following a more prolonged time period post training.

When we carry out a heavy weights session in the gym, training which is predominantly concentric (controlled lifting movements), we will usually feel the fatigue for up to 24 – 48 hours post exercise. However, following a session based largely on eccentric contractions, the fatigue or muscles soreness is not felt until *after* 48 hours and often even later. In the majority of cases, soreness does not dissipate until five days hence.

During stepping, if leading with your left leg, then placing the left foot on the step and then raising yourself up onto it; that movement would consist of a concentric contraction of the left quadriceps. By continuing the motion by leading with the left leg to lower yourself back to the ground then this would constitute an eccentric motion of your right quadriceps as it's this muscle which is controlling the lowering movement. In addition, as the front of the left foot hits the floor, the left calf muscle would be used to eccentrically control the movement of lowering the whole foot flat to the ground. If you don't believe me then try it on a step right now and feel how your toes touch the floor first as your calf muscle controls the lowering of your body.

Therefore, by carrying out a HIIT session involving stepping, these two differing muscles in opposing legs would be feeling the DOMS 48 hours afterwards. It's quite an odd sensation when you have DOMS in this way and one that could result in you walking in circles for a few days.

I took my first dissertation on the effects of post exercise stretching on DOMS and so I know that it's not fully understood why muscle soreness arrives so much later from say stepping than it does with running (unless downhill). But I did discover that (and the existing evidence agreed) post exercise stretching lessened the soreness to a great extent (see below for stretching recommendations). While it did not reduce the amount of time DOMS existed from say 5 days to only 4 – It did reduce the severity of the existing soreness.

If you're an advanced participant, would like to really push yourself and don't mind finding walking a true chore for a while, then upright stepping will be an ideal challenge for you.

Since a good workout balance is always advised, I will also point out that you should alternate leading legs (the front leg carrying out the work) as undoubtedly, the lead leg utilises the muscles in a different way to the trailing leg. Believe me when I say this – You *will* have DOMS following a HIIT session consisting of upright stepping. Instead of having HIIT sessions every other day, as recommended, you'll only be capable of training once every five days. If you don't have much free time then this may well be the right exercise for you, taking everything else into consideration. But in order to add in variety to your workouts, you could always throw in a stepping session once a month or so, at least to try it out.

Swimming

Of course, the HIIT principles still remain intact even when in the water. Swimming has its extreme advocates and flag bearers just like any other HIIT mode.

Swimming carries several advantages that you won't find with the other modes. First – It's low impact and so will be beneficial for those with knee or ankle problems. Second - Swimming will be ideal for those elderly HIIT participants who are perhaps concerned about some of the more high impact modes of training. Third – If you ever find yourself injured then swimming would be the activity that would most likely be recommended due to its low impact nature while the resistance from the water still provides an incredible workout. Indeed when injured, many professional athletes are advised to undertake swimming as part of their rehabilitation.

There are many professional and recreational swimmers who use HIIT protocols in the pool to great effect. While you can of course alter stroke speed in order to increase/lower intensity, emphasis in the pool should always be placed on good form. For that reason, consensus appears to be on altering swim strokes depending on which interval you're presently on. For high intensity intervals then either breaststroke, butterfly or freestyle/front crawl are advised. The latter two strokes in particular are fast paced by nature and therefore naturally vigorous. For recovery periods I suggest using the backstroke as it's slower paced and your face will constantly be out from the water, enabling easier breathing and recovery.

Boxing

I doubt that by now you'll be surprised to learn you can carry out a HIIT workout while boxing. Depending on the kind of day you've had, boxing may even be your preferred choice of workout.

All you need is a heavy bag and some gloves, which by the way I strongly recommend for safety reasons. All gyms will possess these items though purchasing your own pair of gloves may provide you with the extra incentive to give this superb training mode a fair try.

Boxing is ideal for those who may have picked up lower body injuries or who are undergoing rehabilitation anywhere in the lower body.

However, boxing can still be potentially hazardous if correct technique is not utilised. For this reason, I suggest learning proper punching techniques before pounding your fists into a heavy bag at full force. Many health clubs have boxing classes, most commonly Boxercise, but failing that there are hundreds of online videos which demonstrate correct punching techniques. These techniques are often better seen and demonstrated than read about.

There's no need to punch the bag at full force, as simply tapping the bag or punching with medium power is still incredibly intense and carries far less risk of injury. Though feel free to mix in a few hard blows to add variety. And con't forget, you can also add in kicks too. Boxing is a serious workout and so you will feel the burn within seconds.

For recovery periods, it's likely that continuing to punch the bag will be too intense. Instead I suggest jogging on the spot, walking or jogging round the room or light skipping.

Kettlebells

Make no mistake – Kettlebells are back and are becoming extremely popular. Working out with bells can be extremely intense, which of course makes them perfect for us. Most gyms these days have an extensive kettlebell rack.

Like dumbbells, kettlebells come in a range of weights. When performing a HIIT workout using bells for the first time, it's important you don't choose a weight that's too heavy. It's far better to play it safer and go for a lighter weight and then upgrade later, rather than damage your back attempting to swing a weight that's too heavy for you. With bells, we're not going for our 1 rep max. We are instead going for a reasonably sized weight that we can swing with good form, activating a large range of muscle groups in the process.

I guarantee that you'll experience soreness following the first few kettlebell HIIT sessions and naturally this is what you want to try and achieve. But beware of overtraining. If you still feel sore from the last HIIT session then I would suggest refraining from further training until soreness has abated.

There are many exercises you can carry out using kettlebells, but for HIIT purposes it's preferential to use them in a more cardiovascular fashion than simply using them as you would a dumbbell. This means selecting specific exercises that engage as many of the large muscle groups as possible.

Provided below are simple instructions along with a diagram for some of the best kettlebell exercises that fill the HIIT criteria. However, before trying any of these for the first time, I advise further instruction from a qualified gym instructor or at the very least, take a look at a range of explanatory videos online. There are some things that should be seen demonstrated in order to get the feel for correct technique, rather than simply reading about them.

With the majority of exercises in this section – they can be performed with a bell in each hand, one bell in two hands or a single bell in one hand. If you choose the latter then you can alternate hands between intervals. By manipulating these variables as well as the actual weight of the kettlebells themselves, you can constantly make each subsequent training session progressively more intense.

Unlike when doing free weights, with kettlebells, using the momentum is perfectly acceptable. Remember that this is a HIIT workout – The aim is not necessarily to achieve overload in the muscles, but instead to create a heavy build-up of lactic acid.

All movements should be performed in a smooth and fluid fashion. Again, any online training video will show you how they are performed safely and effectively.

With kettlebells perhaps more than with any other training mode, you'll find it convenient to use a timer, HIIT phone app or at the very least a clock to indicate intervals.

I also strongly recommend dynamic stretching (see *Dynamic Stretching*) prior to beginning a HIIT session involving kettlebells.

Clean and Press

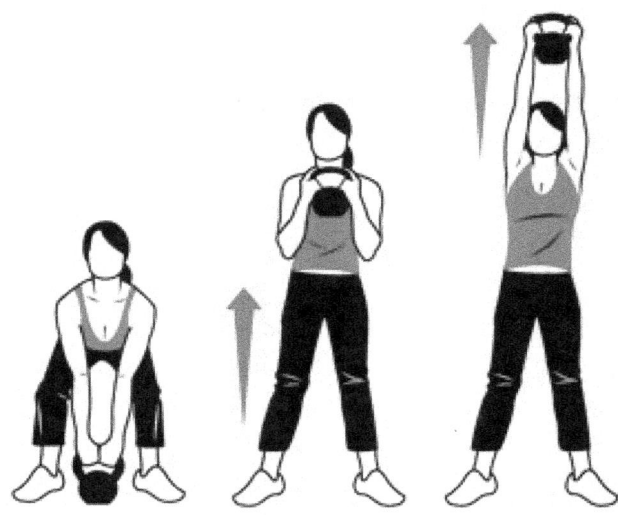

This exercise is carried out in two stages: From the floor to the shoulder and from the shoulder to the overhead position.

Begin in a half squat, taking hold of the bell and with a single clean jerk, pull the weight up to the shoulder. Pause for a beat. Then press the weight above your head. From there, simply allow gravity to assist you in returning the weight back down to the ground. Do not rest the weight on the floor but instead go straight into the next repetition.

Feel free to use the knees to give an extra jerk in order to assist with the raising of the weight during the second stage.

Keep a flat back throughout the entire motion.

Full Swing

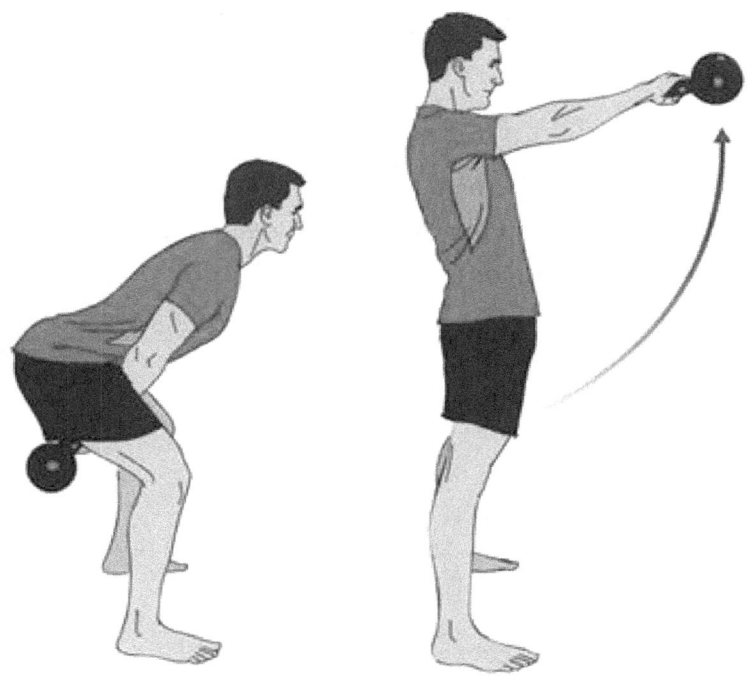

Beginning from a half squat position, swing the bell from between your legs to the arms parallel to the floor position. There is actually the choice of ending the swing motion as the weight is in front of you and your arms are parallel to the floor, or you can continue the motion until it's above your head. Ultimately, the latter will recruit a greater number of muscle fibres to assist with the motion.

The whole manoeuvre is momentum based and uses a great deal of the body's large muscle groups.

As the weight drops down, bend at the knees and hips, going back into a half squat and swing the bell between the legs. As you straighten up, the bell is driven from the legs and body to be carried back to the raised position.

Throughout the motion, the back is kept straight. Try your best to also keep straight arms as you raise and lower the weight. Don't arch your back as the weight reaches the top – Keeping tight abdominals will assist in this.

One Arm Snatch

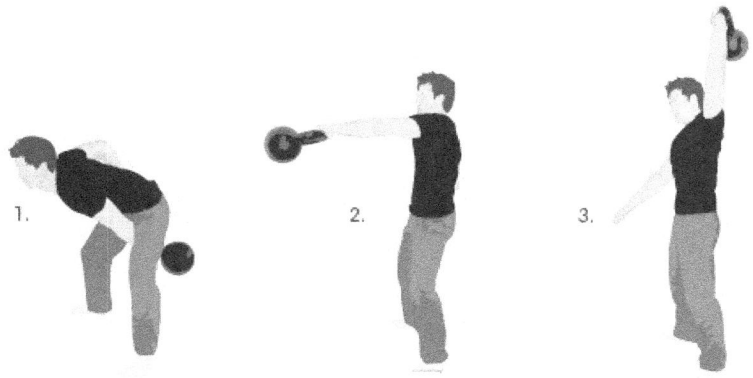

The one arm snatch is a favourite of mine because it utilises nearly every muscle in the body. It's also incredibly fun and there's something just very raw about it.

The one arm snatch should be considered an advancement of the one arm kettlebell swing, so I'd suggest becoming proficient at the above exercise first; with both arms as well as with one since you'll only be using the one arm here.

The difference between the snatch and the swing is that the snatch movement continues until the bell is in the overhead raised position. As usual, swing the bell from between your legs and as the bell raises, lead the motion with your elbow, as if you're about to elbow somebody taller than you in the face. When the bell is in front of your head, simply use a push or spear motion upwards with your arm to raise it to the overhead position. Hold for a beat and then from there, allow gravity to return the bell back to between the legs – Repeat.

The whole motion should be fluid and smooth.

It's important not to hold too tightly onto the weight or it could bang against your forearm in the raised position. A few too many of those and you'll give yourself a bruise.

Figure 8 Curl

This exercise is wonderful for improving coordination and balance as well as strengthening the core muscles. The figure 8 curl is only possible to perform using one kettlebell.

Begin in a half squat and using one hand, pass the weight through your legs and around the back of one knee where your free hand grabs the weight round the other side. From there, bring the weight round the front of your body and curl it up to your chest using a motion identical to a typical bicep curl. Allow the weight to drop down and pass through the legs again. This time, thread the bell round the back of the opposite knee where your free hand will again grasp the handle to bring round the front of your body and again curl up to your chest.

The bell threads between the legs in a figure of 8. The movement is fluid and controlled and should not require any great deal of skill.

As the kettlebell passes between the knees, ensure you bend them slightly along with your hips and use the straightening movement along with the generated momentum to power the curl.

Ensure the back is flat throughout the entire movement.

Squat and Press

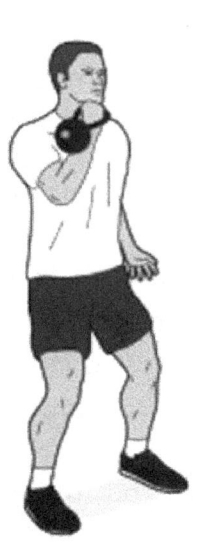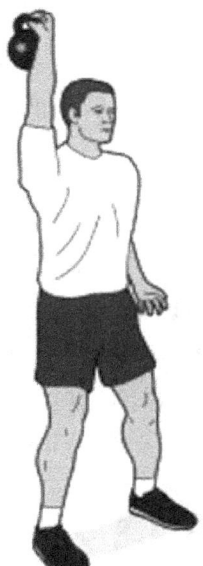

Unlike with the clean and press, with the squat and press the kettlebell remains in the racked position as in the diagram. This exercise works the majority of the body's large muscle groups.

Beginning from a half squat, clean the bell into the racked starting position as shown on the left. Lower yourself into a squat, taking care to go as deep as is comfortable (the deeper you go the more the glutes are incorporated). As you straighten your knees and hips, driving up through the feet, use the momentum to raise the weight above the head in an explosive motion. Control the downward movement of the weight back into the racked position. Then repeat.

Please ensure the bell is returned to the racked position *before* beginning the next squat otherwise the movement could cause you to lose balance.

Lunge and Press

The lunge and press is another exercise that will work a high number of large muscle groups.

Clean the kettlebell up and, if pressing with both hands then hold the weight in front of your chest with both hands. If you're pressing with single arms then clean the weight up into the racked position, ensuring to keep your elbow close into your body.

Lunge forward, bending at the front knee and lowering your rear knee under control towards the floor. As you lower the rear knee toward the floor, simultaneously press the bell straight up and above your head. Complete the manoeuvre by driving up from the front foot while also lowering the weight back toward your chest or racked position.

If pressing with a single arm then always lunge forward with the same leg that is performing the press.

When beginning, this exercise may involve a high level of concentration, skill and balance. It is advisable to begin with extremely light kettlebells. You will benefit from incredible improvements in motor skills by carrying out this exercise on a regular basis.

Keep both feet pointing forward throughout the motion, as well as a straight back and tight abdominals. Don't lunge further forward than is comfortable. If you're not well versed in lunging then please practice the exercise without the press incorporated into it. You can always add the press into subsequent training sessions in order to add another element of difficulty.

Bodyweight Circuits

There are so many different bodyweight exercises that are possible that you'll never find yourself becoming bored with them. However, due to the vast choice available, for HIIT purposes the emphasis should always be placed on selecting those exercises that work the larger muscle groups the hardest. These will predominantly be the legs and core. By selecting exercises that target these areas, you are certain to create a fast lactic acid build up in order to achieve the desired training effect.

These exercises can in the majority of instances be carried out with no equipment. So you can train at home, in the park or in the gym if you choose.

Also, there's nothing stopping you from mixing in these exercises with the above kettlebell exercises for added variation.

These exercises are intense. If doing bodyweight circuits, I highly recommend you pay extra attention to the *dynamic stretching* section below. Many of the bodyweight circuit exercises, particularly the jumping based exercises are by their very nature explosive. Dynamic stretching beforehand will serve you extremely well in preventing any muscle strains during the exercise. The first few times you carry these out, you're going to feel extremely sore for a couple days afterwards. For this reason, I also suggest you pay extra care to carry out static stretches (see *Post*

Workout Stretching) as well as these will partly mitigate the soreness over the following days.

For your recovery periods, you should consider jogging on the spot or around the room, a brisk walk or very light skipping.

Below are a selection of bodyweight circuit exercises along with brief instructions. Select the best few for yourself. As always, if in any doubt, a trainer at your local gym can show you the proper technique. Failing that, there are many online videos available that clearly demonstrate safe and effective technique.

High Knees

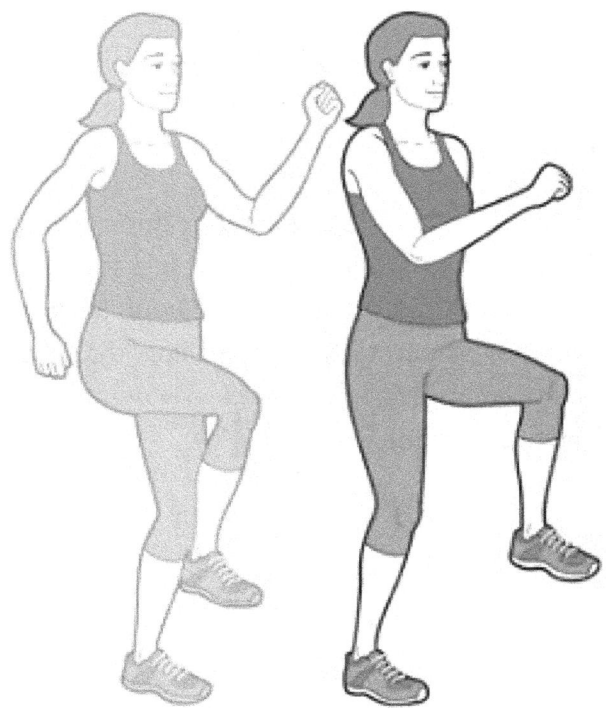

These are an ideal exercise to start with since they are low impact compared to many of the alternatives, therefore they can be treated as part of the warm up before really going all out with the subsequent exercises.

High knees are fairly self-explanatory. The technique is effectively a jogging on the spot movement while concentrating on bringing your knees higher than feels natural.

H gh knees can be made more intense by speeding up the activity while also raising your knees even higher.

Squat Thrusts / Burpees

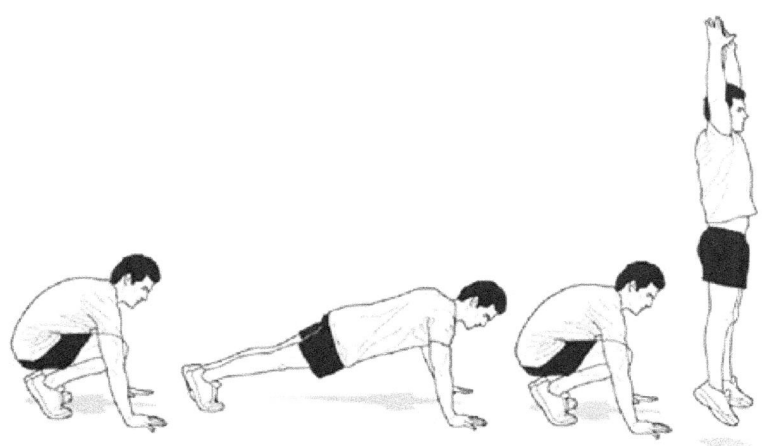

We'll cover both squat thrusts and burpees in this section since there's only one addition from the squat thrust to turn the exercise into a burpee. This exercise works practically every muscle in the body and so will exhaust you quickly.

From a crouched position, place your weight on your hands and shoot your legs straight behind so you end up in the press up position. From here you have the option of adding a press up into the exercise if you choose. Next, shoot your legs back up toward your hands so you're back in the original crouched position. To perform a squat thrust - Simply stand up then crouch back down again and repeat. If you're doing burpees, then instead of simply standing up, jump up into the air in an explosive thrust, stretching your hands up as you do before landing on your feet and returning to the crouch. Repeat.

Squat Jumps

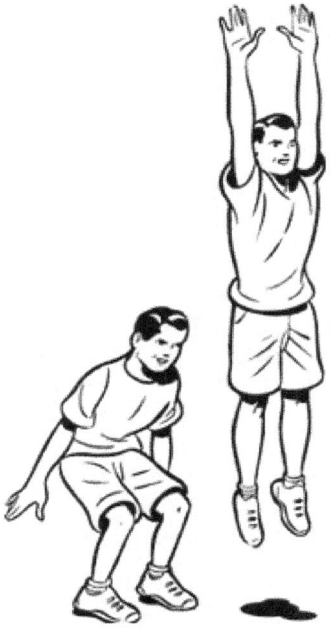

This exercise demonstrates just why dynamic stretching is recommended prior to beginning your session (see section on *Dynamic Stretching* below).

Keep your feet at a shoulder width distance. Control the lowering into the squat and try gain some depth. The more depth you get, the more the powerful glutes are utilised in the explosive movement during the upwards motion. Push through your heels as hard as you can, leaping into the air and stretching your arms to the sky. Keep a flat back throughout and ensure a comfortable landing on the toes.

Many people prefer pointing the arms to the floor as this makes balancing easier. To make the move more advanced therefore, you can point the arms to the sky. You can also concentrate on driving a greater push up through the feet and gaining a higher leap to make the exercise even more intense. It's possible to incorporate a sideward jump into the manoeuvre, jumping wider and wider as you get more used to the variation.

Box Jumping

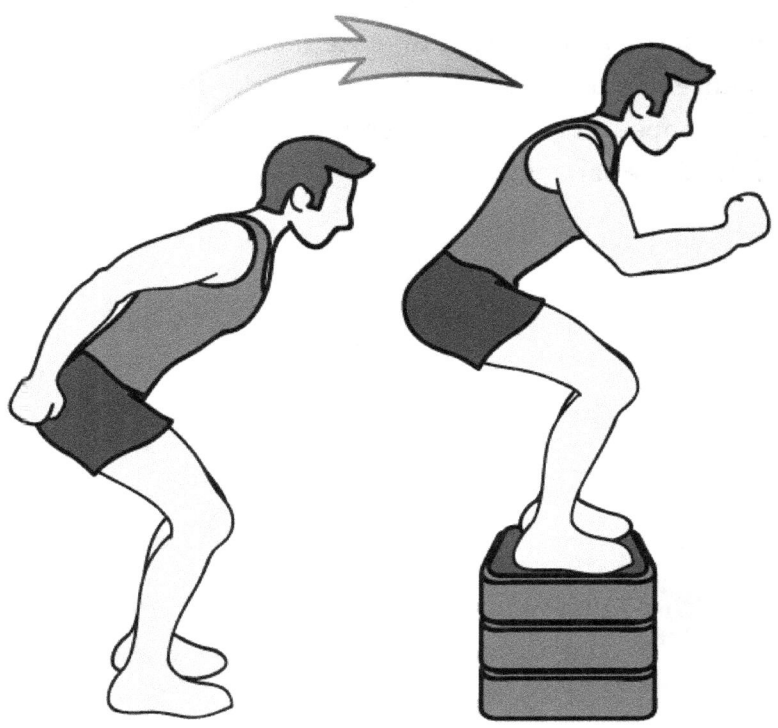

This is one of the few exercises where you need a minimal amount of equipment. All gyms will have boxes which you can stack on top of each other. Otherwise a ledge, bench, high step or suitable wall will work just as well. I know a couple of people who've assembled their own jump boxes using wood from the local DIY store.

With box jumps, you'll find it easier if you don't squat down further than what is necessary. Instead use your arms in a swinging motion to gain momentum for the upward thrust while pushing up through your toes. Bring your knees toward your chest while in the air and keep a flat back.

Once on the box, step up to a fully straightened position, gather your balance for a beat then simply jump backwards the way you came. Repeat.

Keep your knees wide apart (shoulder width) during the entire movement. If you feel them collapsing inwards, then position your feet slightly closer together.

An advanced variation of this exercise is to jump fully over the box, turn around and repeat. You can also carry out the exercise with weights in your hands, which will place even more emphasis on the legs. You can even eliminate the arm swinging motion to force the legs to be even more explosive. Finally, you can raise the height of the box to make the jumps even more intense.

Mountain Climbers

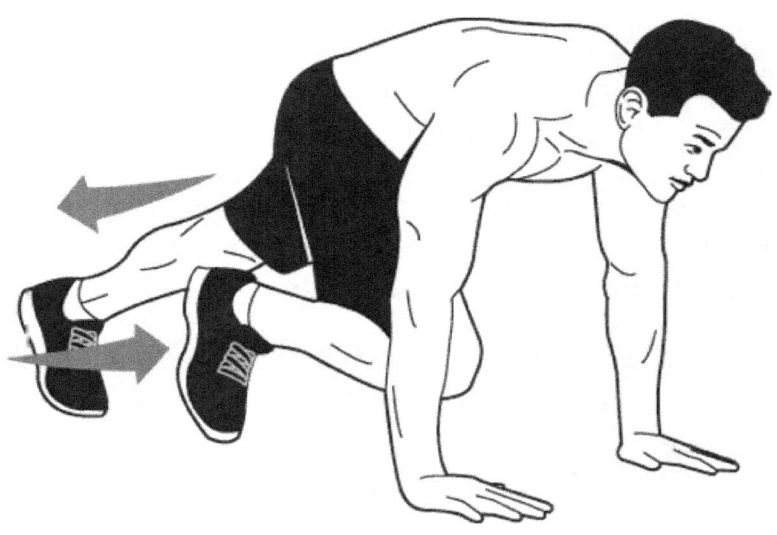

Begin in a peaked push up position with your glutes pointing in the air, placing all weight on your hands. Your arms should be fully vertical throughout the entire exercise with the shoulder fully over the hands. Bring one foot in front of the other so that you're in a comfortable starting position. When ready, switch the position of your legs by utilising a single shifting movement. Repeat again and again in rhythmical fashion. Your hips will bob up and down slightly, which is ok. Once you find your rhythm, feel free to increase the speed to make the exercise more intense.

Concentrate on maintaining a nice breathing rhythm.

Lunge Jumps

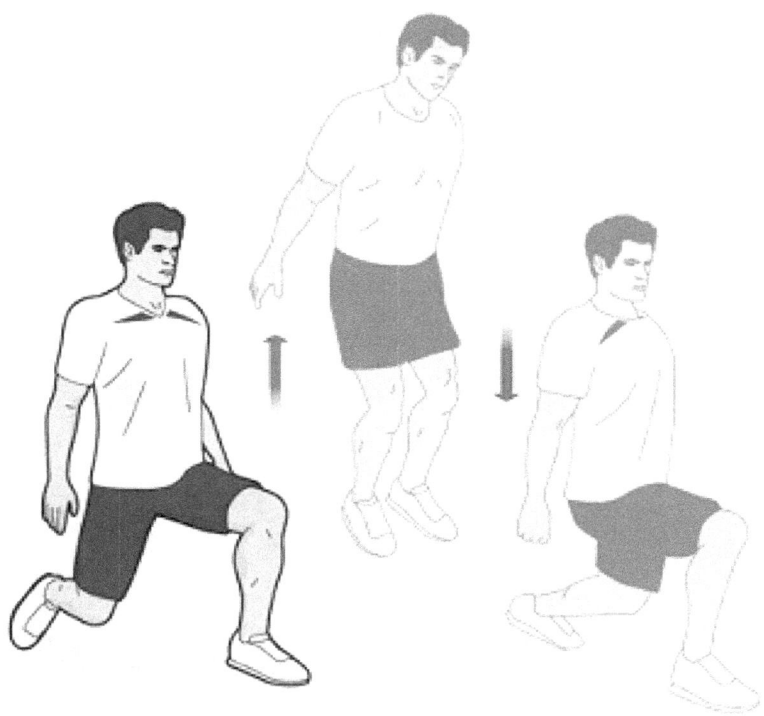

From a standing position, take a large step forward, bending the front knee and dropping the rear knee toward the floor, but not touching it. Jump up through your front foot in an explosive motion and switch legs in mid-air so that your rear leg moves to the front. When the trailing leg reaches the rear, drop the knee toward the floor and repeat.

This move should be carried out on the spot. Ensure you keep a straight back throughout, which should be kept in a straight line above the rear knee.

This exercise is advanced and is excellent for improving balance and coordination. If you feel you lack the balance required then the exercise can be made easier simply by eliminating the leg switching movement. This will still give you an incredible training effect. To make more intense, hold some light weights in your hands.

Tuck Jumps

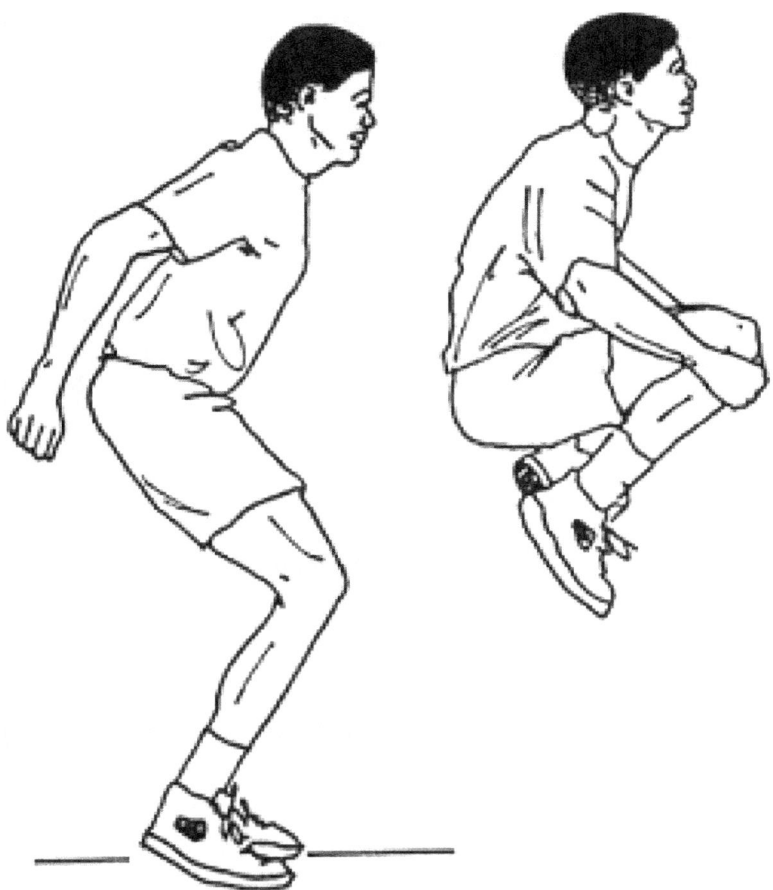

Tuck jumps are similar to squat jumps. The only difference is that this time the aim is to bring the knees in toward the chest before landing. Try and maintain a deep squat just like with squat jumps.

Lateral Box Jumps

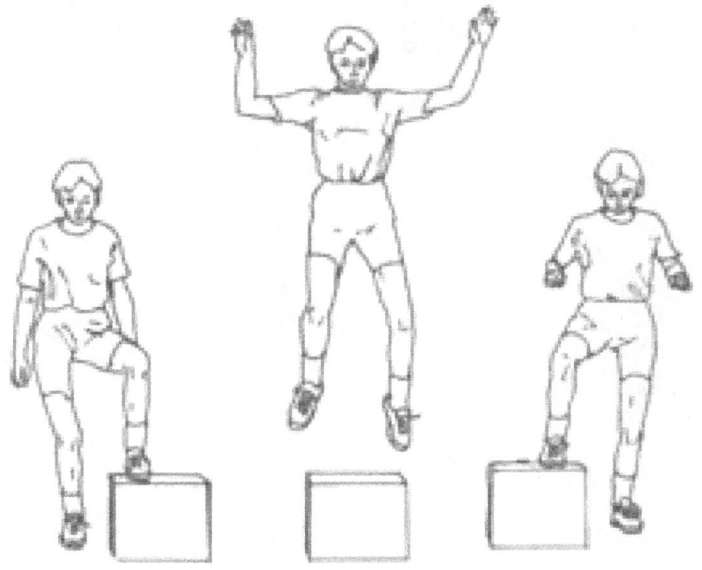

All that's required is a box. There are several variations to this exercise and I hope you'll try them all.

First – Standing to the side of the box, with both feet on the floor, carry out a high jump to the side and landing on top of the box. Jump off the opposite side and repeat in the other direction.

Second – To make the exercise a little harder, you'll be performing a full side jump over the box. Standing to the side of the box, with both feet on the floor, carry out a high jump to the side and fully over the box, landing on the other side. Repeat in the opposite direction.

Third – As in the picture and to make the exercise harder still, you'll be performing the jump using the power from only one leg from a raised position on the box. Push down through the foot of the raised leg in an explosive manoeuvre and land on the opposite side with your other foot on the box ready to take off for the next repetition.

In all exercises you can use your arms to gather momentum and swing yourself over. In the third exercise, you'll find this necessary.

You can make the exercises more intense by raising the height of the box or by speeding up the jumps.

Summary

As you've seen, there are many potential HIIT training modes and within each mode there are modifications you can make in order to increase the intensity incrementally and to ultimately provide a superior training effect, enabling the weight loss to continue without any plateaus.

I understand that most people, myself included, will decide upon their favourite training mode and carry out the vast majority of training within that discipline. Of course that's fine but I'd like you to consider a few points with regards to *cross-training*.

Cross-training refers to training utilising a multi-aspect approach. For example; running on Monday, strength training with weights on Tuesday and swimming on Wednesday would be considered just one example of *cross-training* and is highly recommended for everybody no matter what their training goals may be.

However, keeping in scope with this book, I would like to talk about cross-training with regards to cardio based exercises only – Exercises where we can utilise the HIIT principles.

Each training mode, whether you're doing HIIT or any other training protocol, will utilise specific muscles and nerves in different ways, with different movements, at different frequencies, at different angles, with different ranges of motion at the joints, with a varying degree of force. By carrying out exercise on a bike or rower, you may feel like you're exercising your running muscles, but this will not in fact be giving you the same kind of training as running actually does – Not any more than exercising on a bike or rower would be considered the same kind of training as skipping, swimming or swinging kettlebells.

Each training mode is highly specific. If you don't believe me then simply ask a triathlete if he or she thinks that spending hours in the pool or hours running helps them with their cycling. On the contrary - The interesting element with the triathlon is that by spending time training with either of the three disciplines (swimming, cycling, running), they are actually counteracting what is needed with the other two. Consider that just one training adaptation is the growth of new blood vessels, capillaries in particular which transport fuel, water and oxygen to the working muscles. If you predominantly carry out cycling then the bulk of these new capillaries will be created in the lower extremities. Even though the individual may be considered cardiovascularly fit in an overall context, he may well then have difficulties when switching from cycling to swimming, or from swimming to running.

I'm not telling you this to put you off HIIT cross-training. In fact quite the contrary, I realise the majority of people reading this book will not be triathletes, but I want you to realise there are physiological forces at work that are not yet fully understood and that we should be encouraging partaking in a range of training modes in order to better promote weight loss and at a faster rate.

So with regards to cross-training, let's now consider the overweight teenager, man or woman; the people I wrote this book for.

Though the science is far from definitive, there's a growing body of opinion that agrees that cross-training may be beneficial for a number of reasons.

The American Orthopaedic Society for Sports Medicine says that cross-training can provide a total body tune up. This is something you won't get from only concentrating on one type of activity.

Coming from a common-sense perspective, one can also envisage that cross-training, by randomly selecting from the large selection of HIIT modes above that this would prevent boredom and maintain exercise adherence. Not that HIIT is boring anyway, but you get the idea.

Another benefit is that by exercising a range of muscle groups in different ways alternatively, by choosing different HIIT modes, this may help the individual adapt quicker to new activities. This makes sense. If you're trained in a range of exercise modes then picking up a tennis racket for the first time in your life would be easier for you than if you only ever ran or cycled.

But the primary benefit to cross-training appears to be the reduction in overuse injuries. This is because cross-trainers are not using the same muscles and the same joints in the same way, every time they train.

By spreading the quantity of cumulative stress over a greater number of muscles and joints then individuals can reasonably expect to be able to exercise for longer periods, for greater intensities and much later into their lives. By concentrating on a single activity for years on end, one can expect an increased likelihood of excessively overloading and gradually wearing down vulnerable parts of the body such as the knees, shoulders, hips, ankles, elbows and back. It's important to realise that all cardio exercises, which keep us fit and healthy, utilise repetitive motions of these vulnerable parts. In fact for this very reason, it's even more important for people, once reaching middle-age to cross-train. And this becomes even more crucial still if the individual is particularly prone to injuries or is slow to recover from previous training sessions.

The aim of any training regime, no matter who you are or what your goals may be should be to "shock the body," to create a condition where the body needs to develop, to stress the body in order for it to adapt. By engaging in the same training mode every single time you lace up your training shoes, your body will rapidly become accustomed to the training regime.

Sure you can regularly increase the intensities and ramp up the difficulty of your HIIT protocols, but why not speed up and maximise on your gains by also alternating HIIT modes? By varying HIIT modes regularly you can expect to trigger even faster and more satisfying results, especially when it comes to weight loss.

And in the process, you maximise the chances of remaining fit and healthy, with the capacity to carry out HIIT into the latter stages of your life.

HIIT Best Practices

Before we begin our HIIT session, it's important that our muscles are prepared for the high intensity that's to come. Remember that HIIT is intensive. It's not wise to begin a HIIT session with an all-out sprint. It's far safer to build up to the high intensity periods in a safe, effective and gradual way. Because of this, it's advised that HIIT participants undergo a short pre-workout routine.

Once the session is finished, there should also be a managed, safe and effective post workout routine to ensure a speedier recovery for the next workout.

Below is a checklist of what should be carried out during an entire HIIT session. We'll cover each area now:

- Warm Up
- Dynamic Stretching
- Have A Workout Structure And Target
- Start Low And Build Up
- Ensure Readiness For The Next Interval
- Warm Down
- Post Workout Stretching
- Resting

Warm Up

If I choose to do a HIIT sprint workout in the local park, then it's a 7 minute walk from my front door. This walk is an essential part of my warm up.

As soon as I arrive at the park, I begin a slow jog. This jog lasts for around 3 minutes until I reach the track. I have a tree which marks the spot where I begin my dynamic stretching routine (see immediately below).

By this point I've had a nice gradual warm up, oxygenated blood is already flowing at a faster rate around my body ready to give energy and oxygen to my muscles when the real work begins. If the blood is not already flowing at an increased rate when I begin my high intensity intervals then oxygen and energy cannot get to where they're needed quick enough. This is why you tire out and fatigue quickly when you don't warm up.

To reiterate – If you work at 100% intensity without having gradually increased your heart rate, then you will not have adequately prepared your heart and lungs to deliver oxygenated blood to your muscles, which in turn will not have been prepared to receive it. This will result in a sluggish training session where you'll be performing far below your capabilities.

A warm up also oils your joints in preparation for the work ahead. It does this by distributing synovial fluid, a natural lubricant. This will help prevent an injury.

Warming up enhances the transmission of nerve impulses, helping you think, act and react quicker. This is the reason you don't think clearly when you just wake up, because your nerves are cold.

While it's perhaps best as well as most convenient to warm up using a mode specific to the impending HIIT session, it's not absolutely essential. If the HIIT workout is sprinting, then jogging is the obvious warm up. If cycling, then an easy cycle with low resistance is obvious since you'll already be sat on the bike. Likewise with rowing or any other mode you choose. Moving the muscles, the legs in particular in a way specific to the approaching workout makes complete sense for reasons of specificity.

If you're carrying out a kettlebell or bodyweight circuit session then yes, it is possible to carry out the forthcoming exercises with less intensity, using lighter weights and without incorporating a full range of motion – A half squat with no weights for example. But my personal preference would be to utilise a treadmill, rower or cycle ergometer rather than an easier version of bodyweight circuits.

Once the warm up has been completed, then move quickly on to some dynamic stretching.

Dynamic Stretching

Remember physical education or gym classes back at school when you used to always carry out a bunch of static stretches before the real work began? Well this is an example of an unnecessary practice that is in the national psyche simply through habit. Not only is a pre-workout static stretch not necessary, it is actually potentially dangerous.

To clear up any confusion, static stretches are the most commonly used stretches that are held at a point of tension for around 10 – 15 seconds. We have been using them all our lives.

The reason we were always made to do static stretches pre-workout was to prevent injury. That was the only reason. However, studies have shown that there are no differences to the level of injuries sustained during the subsequent activity between groups that carry out pre-workout static stretches and those that don't.

In fact by giving cold muscles static stretches before your workout has even begun, you are in fact more likely to be injured during or after the activity than if you don't stretch. It's far easier to tear a cold muscle than a warmed up muscle due to it being less malleable. So you really don't need to bother wasting your time carrying out pre-workout static stretches, and that goes for the rest of your life, it's just not necessary.

However, *dynamic stretching* is another matter entirely. Dynamic stretches use controlled movements in order to improve range of motion, loosen up the muscles, increase the heart rate and body temperature as well as the blood flow around the body. In fact, incorporating dynamic stretching at this point in your HIIT session can be considered an extended part of your warm up.

Dynamic stretching is most effective when used prior to activities that involve explosive movements. For HIIT purposes, this would most likely encompass sprinting and jumping, though explosive bursts are possible in a range of other HIIT modes too. No matter what your present physical condition and no matter what your future goals may be (once you've achieved your dream weight) – If you are utilising explosive body movements in your HIIT workouts, which I accept will be the case in the vast majority of instances, then I recommend you incorporate dynamic stretches into your sessions.

Dynamic stretching is used to its best effect when the movements are kept specific to the upcoming activity. For sprints you would mimic sprint movements and for jumps you would mimic jumping movements etc.

The idea is to start slowly, using a small range of motion and focusing on good form. After a set number of repetitions (usually a small number) and you feel the movements becoming easier, then you would gradually increase the range of motion as well as speed. The key is to keep the movements dynamic. At the further points of the larger movements made, the muscles are being stretched for a brief second (dynamically) and in a manner that will soon be occurring during the chosen activity.

For HIIT sprint and jumping workouts, particular emphasis should be placed on the hamstrings; a common area of straining.

There is no requirement to spend a great deal of time carrying out dynamic stretches. You should spend only the amount of time required to bring your joints through the greater ranges of motion, thus stretching the muscles, for a small number of repetitions. Once you reach your full range of motion, ten repetitions are usually enough for most people to have dynamically stretched the targeted muscles. Although you should always use your own best judgement and listen to your body. There are many factors at play that could affect your state on the day and therefore how many repetitions you should carry out. Temperature, weather, surface, hydration, alertness, mood and time of day can all play a part and affect your flexibility at any given time. If in doubt, it's always preferential to carry out a few extra repetitions than too few and risk straining a muscle because you performed explosive movements on cold muscles that hadn't been fully mobilised and stretched.

As you may have already guessed, I'm a fan of getting in there and getting out. I like to get the greatest benefits from my workouts in the shortest possible time period. If you would prefer to spend more of your time carrying out an extended warm up (that was specific to your HIIT mode) then there will be a gradually diminished need to spend more time dynamic stretching. Likewise the same goes for the opposite – Since dynamic stretching utilises large movements of the body, which in some instances are quite intense as you're about to discover, if you would rather spend more time dynamic stretching, you can choose to shorten your warm up. As always, listen to your body and never go all out 100% for your high intensity interval until you're satisfied you are thoroughly prepared.

Now we'll take a look at a range of specific dynamic stretches.

Pike Stretch

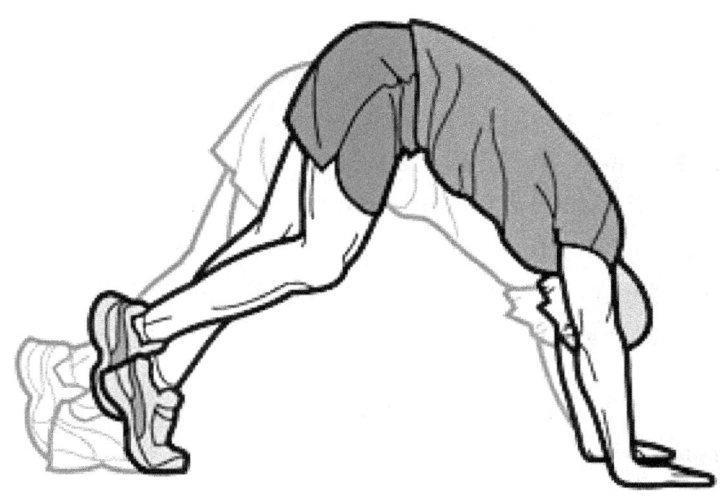

Target Muscles – Calf Muscles

I recommend beginning with the pike stretch since it's the least energetic of all the dynamic stretches we'll be covering. By starting with this one, you'll be able to build up to the more intense stretches below.

Begin with your hands and knees on the floor, then raise your hips into the air so your body is in the piked position as in the drawing. Take one foot from the ground and place it on the heel of the active (to be stretched) foot. Push down with your free foot so the heel of the active foot presses toward the ground. Hold for a second and release. Repeat.

If you're particularly flexible then you may not require the use of your free foot for pressing down the active foot.

To increase the intensity of the stretch, slide the feet further away from your hands. If you weren't already, you can also ensure your heel presses all the way to the ground.

Butt Kicks

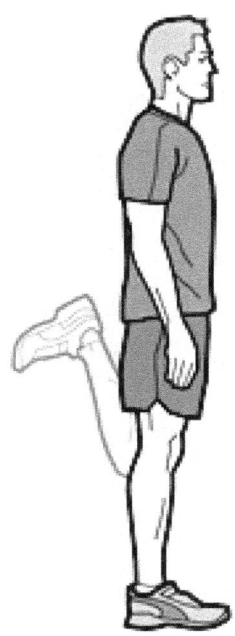

Target Muscles – Quadriceps

Stand tall and walk forward with an exaggerated back kicking motion with your heels moving toward your glutes. Increase the intensity by advancing to a slow jog, kicking higher and faster.

Leg Swings

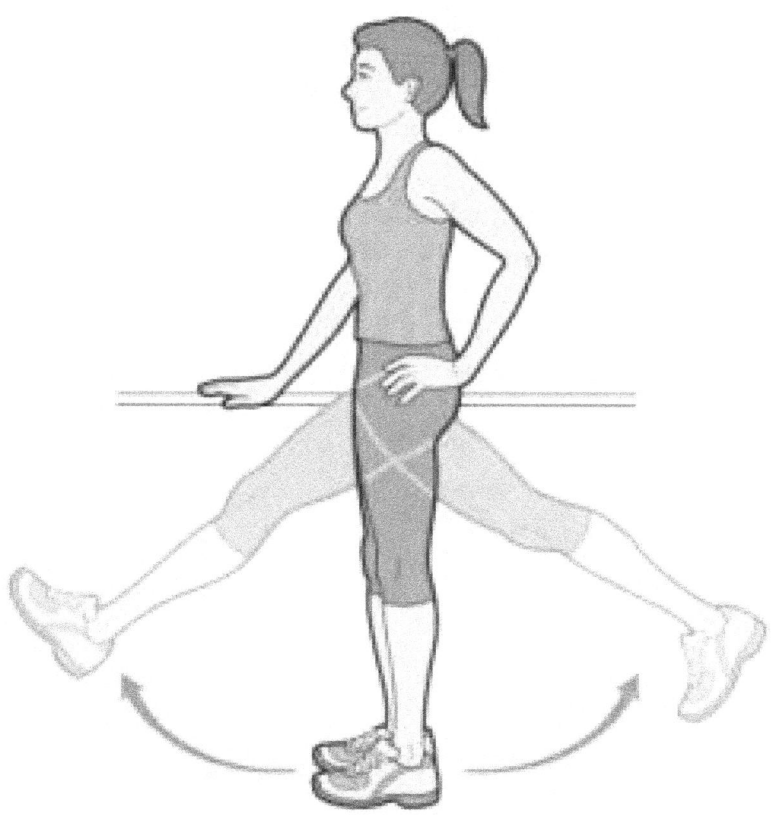

Target Muscles – Hip Flexors, Glutes, Hamstrings

Best used with a wall, tree or rail as a support.

The forward swing stretches the glutes and hamstrings, whereas the backward swing stretches the hip flexors.

The knees should be soft and not locked out. In fact the emphasis with the forward swing portion of this exercise should be placed on the glutes which means you don't need to be too concerned with keeping your knee overly straight – Hamstrings are secondary here and this provides a nice warm up for the straight leg raises (hamstrings) later on. During the backward phase of the swing, the knees will naturally bend regardless.

Begin slow with a small range of motion. Increase the intensity by speeding up the movement and increasing the range of motion.

Straight Leg Raises

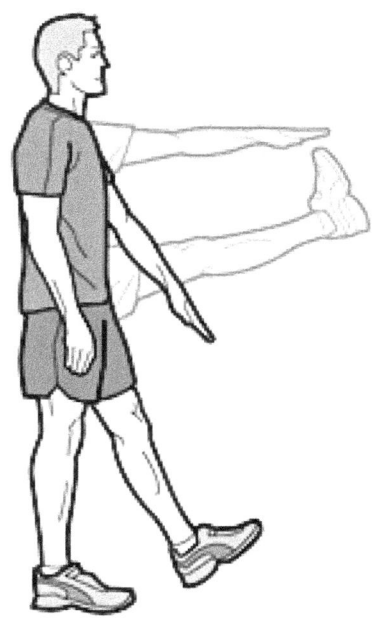

Target Muscles – Hamstrings, Calf Muscles

Unlike the compound stretch above, here we are primarily stretching the hamstrings, a crucially important area for dynamic stretching prior to sprinting or jumping.

Maintain a straight posture as you walk forward lifting your legs in the air. Ensure your knee remains as straight as possible as bending it in any way will shorten rather than lengthen the hamstrings which we are targeting here. By pointing the toes toward your head, the calf muscles will also be dynamically stretched. Look straight forward while carrying out the exercise as this will aid balance.

To advance this exercise, simply increase the speed or add a skipping motion instead of walking. The legs can also be raised higher.

Walking Lunges

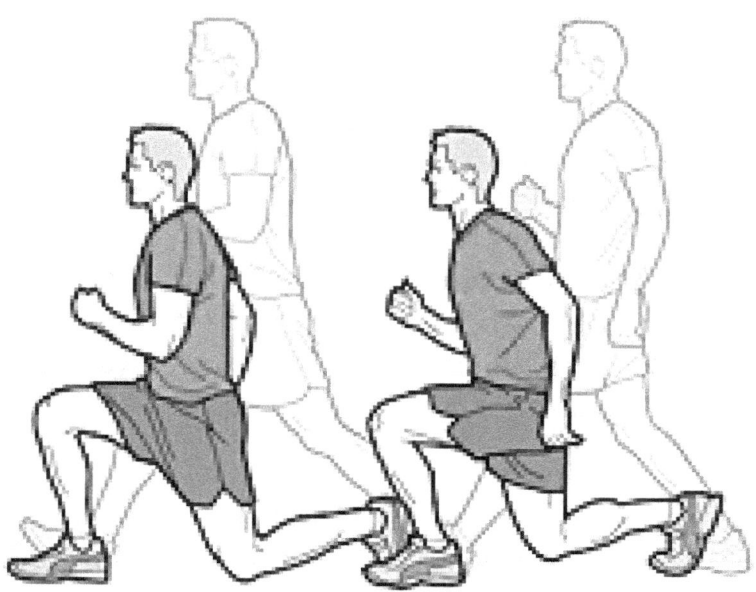

Target Muscles – Hip Flexors, Hamstrings, Quadriceps, Calf Muscles

Walking lunges are a mini-workout in themselves. For this reason they should be put at the end of your dynamic stretching routine when you'll be most warmed up and ready to begin your high intensity intervals.

This dynamic stretch also involves all the running muscles including the glutes if a slight modification is made.

Place your hands on your hips and step forward with one foot. Bend your front leg as you lower your back leg to the ground in a controlled manner. The front knee should not extend beyond the point of the toes and you should not allow your rear knee to touch the ground. Your body weight should be centred over the front leg and you use the same foot to push back up to a standing position. Now step through with your rear foot thus changing sides. Keep an upright posture throughout, pulling in your abdominals.

In order to add a stretch to your glutes - As you bring your rear leg forward, first raise the knee (of the rear leg) up to your chest. Clasp at the knee using both hands and pull the knee into your chest. You should feel the stretch in your glutes. Bring the leg down in front, going into your next lunge. This is in effect incorporating a standing knee raise to your lunges.

By now you should be thoroughly warmed-up, dynamically stretched and ready to begin your high intensity intervals. But remember to use your own best judgement. It may be an extremely cold day and if you're exercising outside, then you can always go back into a warm up and build up to the high intensity intervals.

Have A Workout Structure And Target

It would be beneficial to enter your training session with a HIIT plan in your head and therefore some sort of idea of any targets within that session. For example; how many high intensity intervals are you hoping to squeeze in? Will it be one more than during the previous workout? Will the high intensity periods be more intense or will the recovery periods be shorter?

I always like to know exactly what the coming workout has in store for me, then if I don't achieve my goals, I can beat myself up over it and make sure I achieve them the time after. I do this by analysing where I went wrong – Was I not properly hydrated? Did I not get enough sleep? Were the intervals too tough for me? Or was I just having a bad day?

I would also suggest making a record of your achievements at the end of your workout. The following could be useful; number of intervals, duration of high intensity periods, duration of recovery periods, HIIT mode.

By keeping a record of the above variables, improving on each subsequent training session can be an attainable target. If you intend on regularly alternating HIIT modes then it could be a while before returning to say rowing and remembering exactly how well you did on your previous session could be tricky.

Getting more specific - Let's take the example that you'll be carrying out HIIT running outside in the park, but feel free to modify accordingly depending on your chosen activity. I have to use some sort of an example here and I've chosen running outside as it's genuinely very popular.

It would be best to have a predetermined route planned out. So why not take a walk along your chosen path the day before your first session. Mark out where you'll begin your walk, where you'll start your light jog and your marker (tree, lamp post, trash can) for your first high intensity interval.

Then mark out the spot where this sprint will end and your recovery period will begin. This recovery period should be quite lengthy when starting out, maybe even up to 3 minutes in duration so have this pre-planned. Then locate your next landmark for your next high intensity interval.

I've found that this is so much easier if you have a circuit, such as a track around the outside of a park then you can use the same markers on each lap as your cue to change speed.

Of course, you can bypass using any markers at all if you simply choose to listen to your own body in the moment and change speeds/intensity accordingly. There is no problem in doing this as long as you can honestly say to yourself that you did reach the magic 100% maximum intensity level, if only for a few seconds.

Start Low And Build Up

You need to think about your existing level of fitness.

Are you immediately ready to go for a full on HIIT session consisting of between 8 – 10 high intensity periods with only very short recovery periods? Or is your present fitness level a little more modest and you're in need of working up to the former?

Everybody has to start somewhere so don't fret if you're nervous about putting this book down and starting your first HIIT session.

If you're fit and confident, then you may as well dive straight in at the deep end and see how you get on with it. There's no way any number of all-out sprints interspersed with recovery periods will phase or harm you. Just make a note of your variables and try to advance yourself on the subsequent sessions.

For those starting with modest fitness, then this section is a little more for you.

If you're beginning from an extremely low cardio base, then I suggest taking at least two continuous training sessions first. If you're able to run, cycle, row etc for 30+ minutes at 70% of your maximal heart rate, then in my opinion, you're perfectly fine to begin HIIT sessions. Your initial HIIT sessions should encompass high intensity periods of shorter duration coupled with longer recovery periods.

From a relative warm up intensity such as walking or light jogging, then injuries permitting, anybody no matter who they are will be able to increase the intensity to something higher than the warm up state. Bingo - Because as soon as you've done this, then as long as you return to a lower intensity then this can be considered interval training.

If your recovery intensity is 50 – 60% maximal heart rate (achievable for everybody) then raising that to 70 – 85% will be manageable by everybody too.

If you're intending on taking it easy during the first session, then 4 high intensity periods, at 30 seconds each will give you a feel for what it's all about. Judge for yourself, in the moment, how long the recovery periods should be and then take the next high intensity intervals when ready. All I do ask is that you record the variables and endeavour to smash them on each subsequent training session. Trust me, there's no better feeling than improving just that little bit with each subsequent training session and while you're still discovering exactly where your fitness or HIIT level is then these original *improvements* will come thick and fast. It's similar to beginning a strength training regime - Until you know what you're capable of lifting then there'll be much experimentation until you find the correct weights, with each exercise that you're capable of lifting between 6 – 8 times until you reach overload.

Though I will reiterate this here, as I have several times already – It's all about intensity. And I urge you to push yourself and see just what you're capable of achieving, rather than playing it safe. You may just surprise yourself.

Ensure Readiness For The Next Interval

Remember that a crucial part of HIIT is the recovery period. Don't assume that just because you're walking or cycling at an easy intensity and you're finding the intensity to be extremely easy that you're somehow not doing HIIT correctly. The recovery period is just as important as the high intensity period. The walks are just as important as the sprints. The cycling on minimal resistance is just as important as cycling on high resistance.

So ensure your recovery periods are sufficient enough to bring your heart rate down to a more relaxed state and your body feels prepared for the next high intensity interval. Throughout your HIIT session there'll be several high intensity-intervals that if you don't feel shattered after your first or second, you will do by the time you get to your fourth of fifth, eleventh or twelfth.

So enjoy the recovery periods and make full use of them. They're also the best opportunity you'll have to take a gulp of water – Which I recommend you do often.

Warm Down

Just as warming up at the beginning of a HIIT session is crucial, so is warming down at the end. This is something that many people don't know the significance of and the effects of not warming down can be debilitating.

When you exercise, you are increasing the flow of blood around your body. So if you exercise hard, and then come to a sudden stop, although you and your muscles have stopped working, your blood will still be flowing at this increased rate. Because of gravity, your blood will tend to pool in your legs. If blood is pooled sufficiently so that there's a reduction in return flow to the heart then your blood pressure can drop and you will become dizzy or possibly even faint. I'm sure you're aware of the feeling of having heavy legs after a run, maybe even for a couple of days afterwards? This could have been due to not warming down properly and experiencing the subsequent blood pooling.

By gradually lowering the intensity of your HIIT session then you can safely bring your heart rate back down to a more regular pace.

The way I do this is that after I've finished my final high intensity period, instead of walking like I would a usual recovery period, I will instead lightly jog for a couple of minutes. Afterwards I will continue with a walk for a few minutes after that.

This way my heart rate has been gradually returned to a more normal pace, even though my blood is still circulating in a high gear, my legs are still moving too.

Never will I collapse on a bench after an all-out sprint.

Post Workout Stretching

I mentioned "heavy legs" in the section above; the feeling of not being able to move your legs the day or two after your workout. This feeling can be prevented by warming down as we've already discussed and also by carrying out a thorough post workout stretch.

When you carry out exercise, you are contracting your muscles, often with extreme force. Contracting is another word for shortening. If you don't stretch your muscles after you've been repeatedly shortening them during your workout then trust me, you'll know about it in the morning as you'll feel extremely stiff. You need to bring your muscles back to their pre-workout length by stretching them.

Post workout would also be a good time to try and *improve* your flexibility, by stretching perhaps a little deeper and for longer. These types of stretches are known as *developmental stretches* as they work on increasing your flexibility and not merely returning your muscles to their original length. Post workout is the safest and most effective time to carry out developmental stretches since you'll be thoroughly warmed up and your muscles will be the most pliable. If you follow the advice in this book, then you will be carrying out a lot of HIIT sessions and so developmental stretches should be a regular part of your post workout routine as they will help to improve your posture, decrease the chances of muscle cramping and will even lessen the chances of injury. The most common form of injury sustained by sprinters are hamstring strains and so developmental stretches which target the hamstrings are particularly important.

Developmental stretches are similar to the usual static stretches we've been using all our lives. With a static stretch, the stretch is held for around 10 – 15 seconds at a point where the tension is felt. At the point in time where you feel the tension diminish - the stretch is developed further by going deeper into it and holding the position for around 30 seconds. As you sink further into the stretch, breathe out gently through your mouth. Once you feel the tension diminish once again, you can then go even further into the stretch. As you go deeper into the stretch, ensure you do so in a slow and controlled manner. Remember that the idea is to *feel* the tension otherwise you are not actually stretching the muscle. If you feel the tension too much so that it becomes uncomfortable then ease yourself out a little until it feels more bearable.

You should carry out a range of stretches on all the major muscles of the legs as well as the upper body, as don't forget, we also use the arms a great deal while running and using other modes of HIIT. While you can perform developmental stretches on any muscle, I feel the most important area for HIIT purposes are the hamstrings which also happens to be an area where too many people suffer from inflexibility. I will reiterate - It is advisable to at least carry out static stretches on all the main muscle groups immediately after your warm down. But if you decide to only carry out developmental stretches in one area, then this area should be the hamstrings.

Below are diagrams as well as instructions for carrying out a range of important stretches – beginning with the hamstrings, although please feel free to skip this part if you're fully aware about how these stretches are carried out. Explanations on how to develop each stretch further will also be given. In most instances, I give two variations of each stretch and you should carry out the stretch you prefer and feel you're getting the most benefit from. However, as always, alternating your stretches every few HIIT sessions will provide additional benefits.

Lying Hamstring Stretch

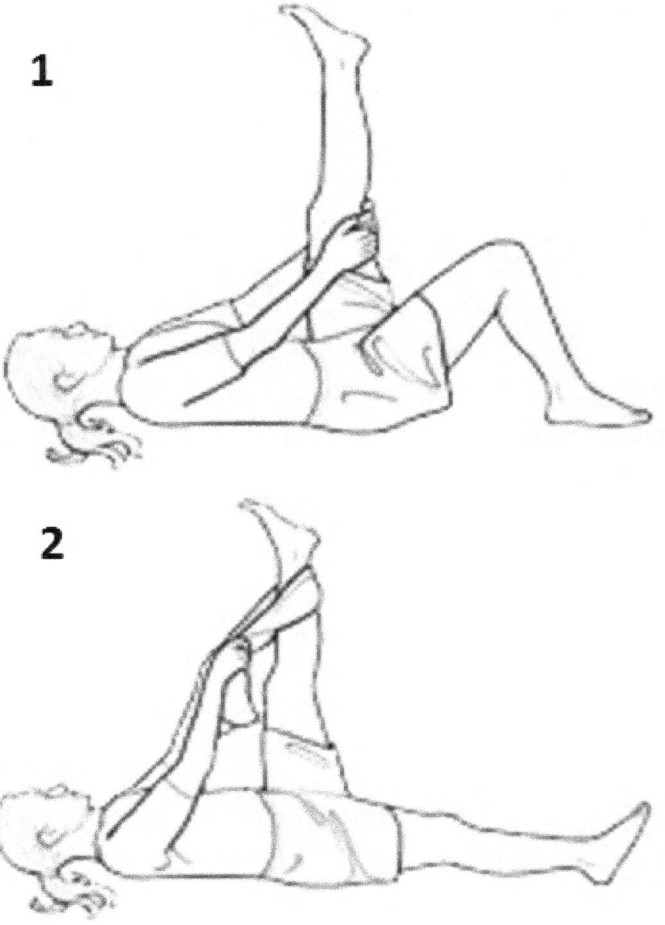

1. The lying hamstring stretch is carried out on each leg individually. Lie down with your back flat on the ground and raise one leg, taking hold behind the knee with your hands.

2. By bending the knee of your free leg you'll take pressure off your back.

3. Gently pull the leg towards yourself until you feel the stretch.

4. Ensure you keep the knee as straight as possible but not locked. You will feel a natural tendency to bend the knee, which will lessen the stretch – Try and avoid that.

5. If you're developing hamstring flexibility as suggested then when tension is no longer felt (20 – 30 seconds), ease the leg closer toward your chest until you feel new tension.

6. Repeat as necessary and then change legs.

7. Image 2 shows the use of a towel which may be used if you can't reach your knee.

Standing Hamstring Stretch

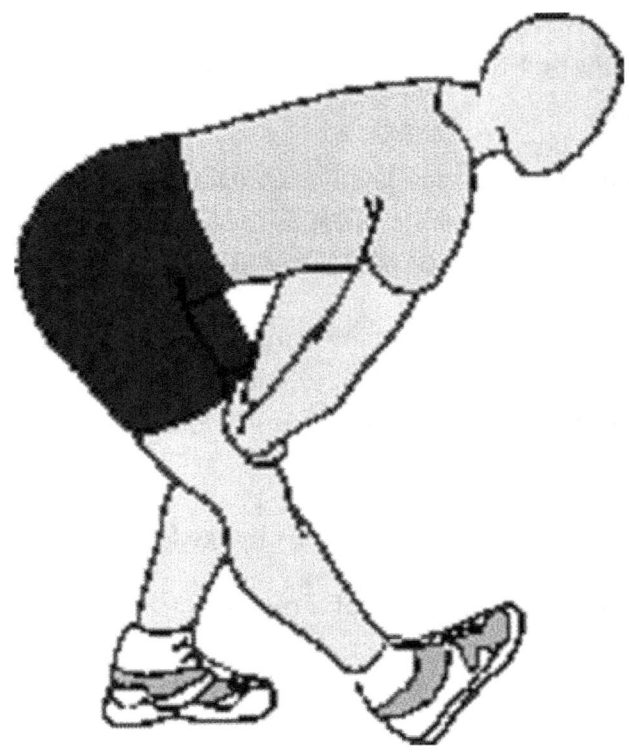

I'm sure the vast majority of people reading this book are familiar with this stretch. The standing hamstring stretch will yield the same results as the above lying hamstring stretch except by raising the toes of the leg being stretched, you can also gain a stretch on the calf muscles.

In order to develop further, simply lower your chest further toward the straightened leg, ensuring to keep the knee straight but not locked and your back straight. You can also slide the foot in closer toward your bent leg to deepen the stretch.

Standing Quadriceps Stretch

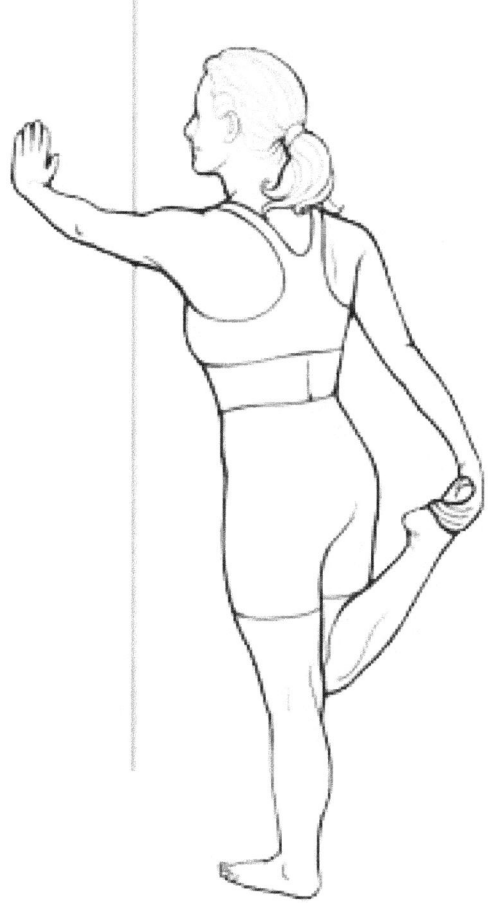

Balance yourself against a wall with one hand. Use your other hand to clasp the foot or ankle of the corresponding leg. Pull your foot toward your glutes until you feel the stretch in your quadriceps. You can increase this stretch by pulling your foot even closer to your glutes. If you're not feeling a deep enough stretch then try the method below.

Hip Flexor / Quadriceps Stretch

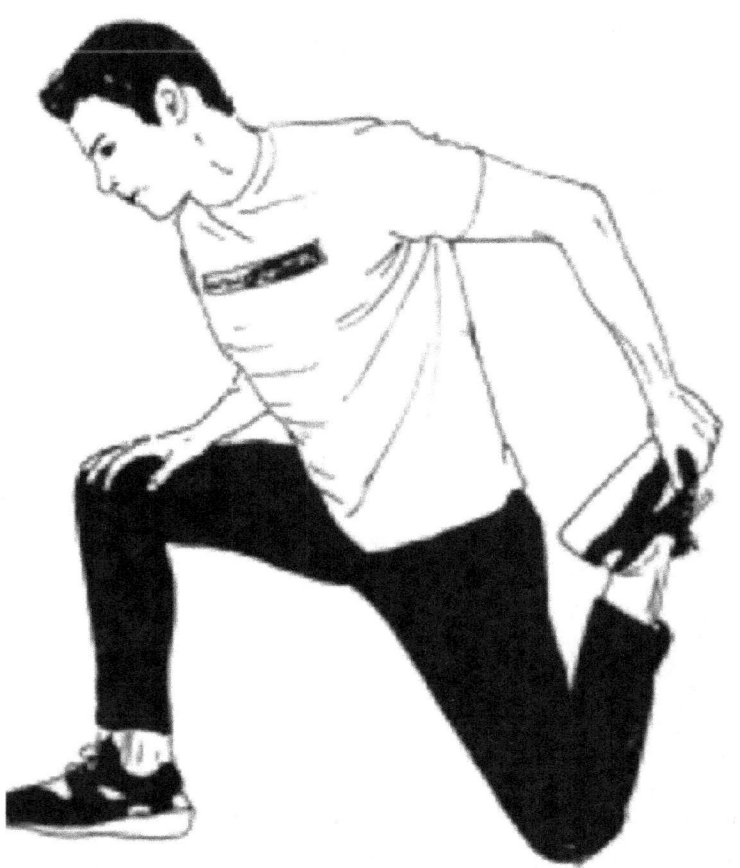

I will warn you that this stretch is deep. But it gets the job done. Not only does this stretch out your quadriceps extremely well, but also your illopsoas muscles which are the strongest of your hip flexors.

Kneel on the floor with one knee in front of the other. Bend the knee of your rear leg and clasp your foot with the corresponding hand. This may require balance so you may use a chair or wall to stabilise yourself. Be careful not to place too much weight on the knee – Leaning forward will take the weight off or you can place a towel between the knee and the floor. Once you're in position, simply push out your hips to feel the stretch in your hip flexors and quadriceps. You can develop the stretch by pushing your hips out further or by stepping forward gradually with your front foot.

Calf Stretch

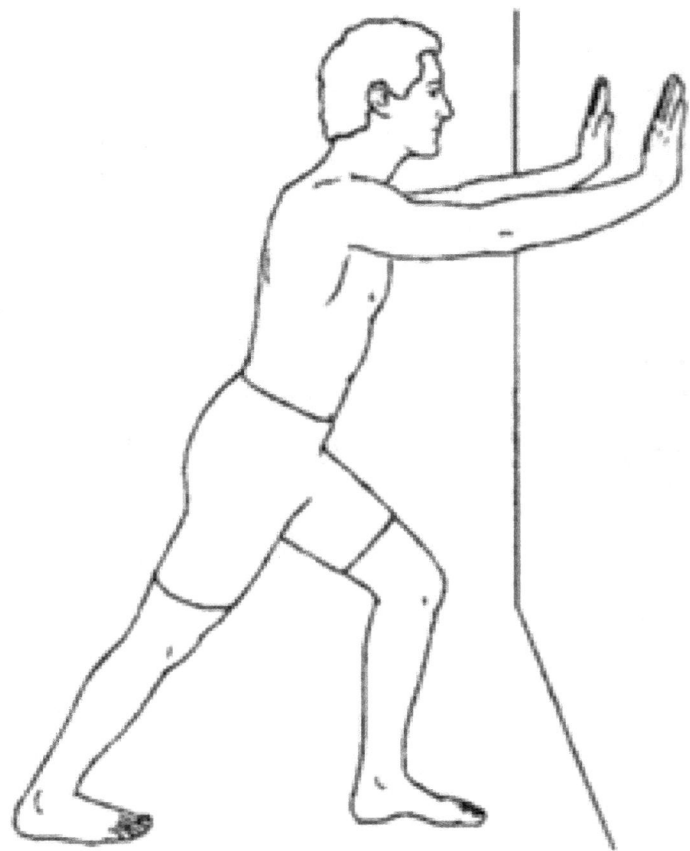

This is the classic calf muscle stretch I'm sure you've been using since you were a child. While you don't require a wall as illustrated in the drawing, using one will enable you to maintain a better balance. Ensure both feet point forwards and keep your rear foot flat against the floor. By sliding back the rear foot you decrease the angle between the toes and the shin, gradually lengthening the muscle in the back of the leg and increasing the tension of the stretch. Your rear heel may feel the natural tendency to rise up from the ground, but it's important to keep it flat. As with all developmental stretches, when you feel the tension wane, gradually increase the tension (in this case by sliding the rear foot further back) and hold for another 30 seconds.

Soleus Stretch

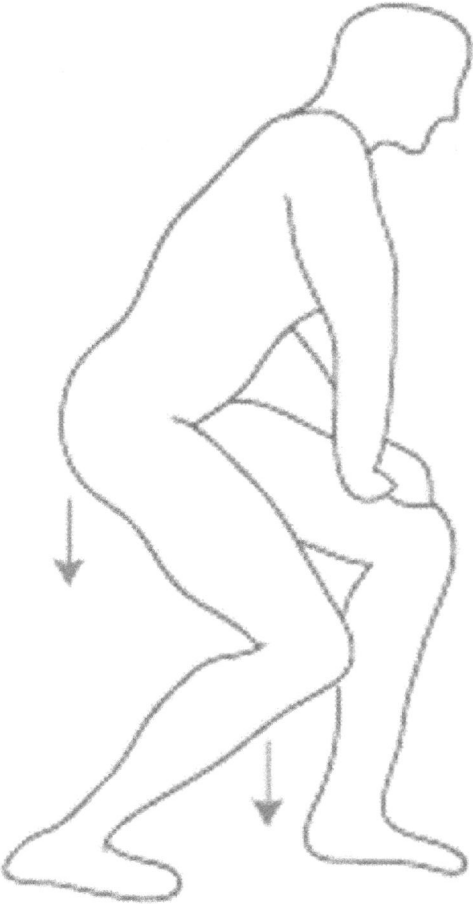

The soleus muscle runs deeper to the calves and connects to the heel. Many runners often find the soleus becomes tight, causing discomfort and it's thought that a tight soleus muscle may also be a contributing factor toward Achilles tendonitis. Despite this, it's not an area we often stretch, probably because we were never taught how to do it. Yet stretching the soleus is used as a preventative measure from Achilles tendonitis.

To carry out this stretch, the angle of the ankle joint between the toes and shin must be reduced. Unlike when stretching the calves however, when stretching the soleus, the knee is bent, in order to take the calf out of the stretch.

As in the diagram, the front leg is used for stabilisation. Bend the rear knee, ensuring you're narrowing the angle of the ankle joint. You'll feel the stretch at the back of your leg just above the heel.

To develop this stretch, simply lower your thighs closer to the ground as in the diagram, thus further decreasing the angle of the ankle joint.

This stretch is deep. I suggest you come out from the stretch slowly.

Alternative Soleus Stretch

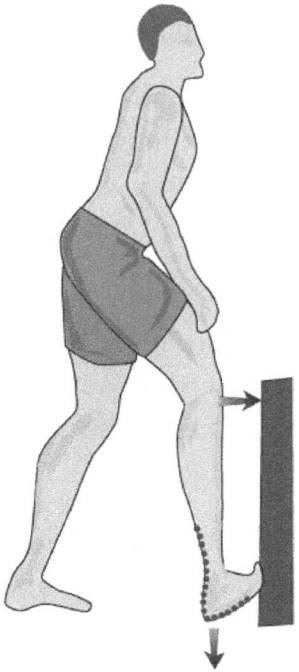

As an alternative to the above, you can simply use a wall, lamp post or pillar/post at the gym to stretch the soleus.

Plant the heel on the floor with your toes reaching upward against the wall for support. Move your knee towards the wall, thus reducing the angle at the ankle and stretching the muscle.

To develop further, simply move your knee closer to the wall.

This is a deep stretch that you will *feel*. When finished, ensure you relax out from it slowly.

Triceps Stretch

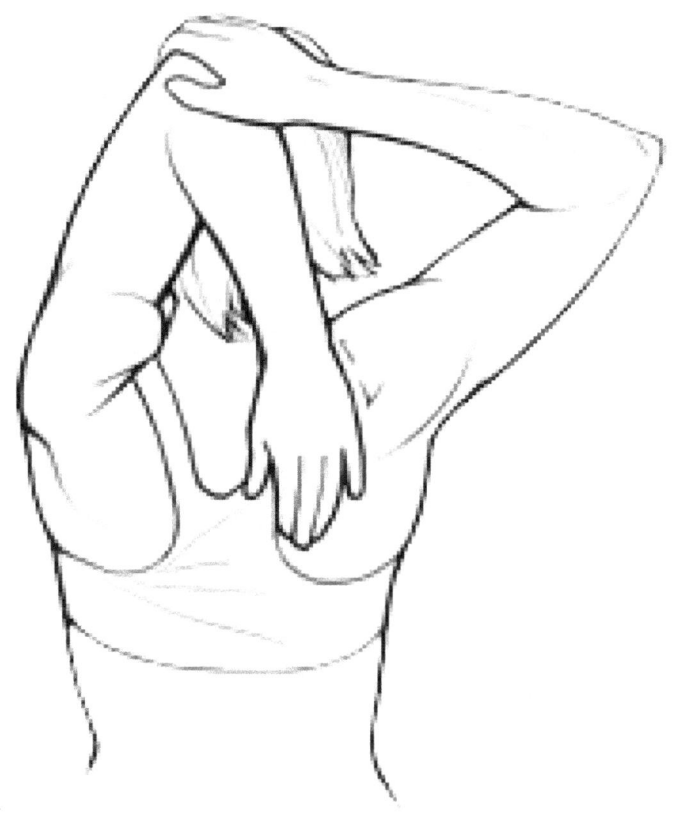

We need to also incorporate a number of upper body stretches in order to promote all over flexibility and good health. Let's not forget that we also use our arms when performing a large range of HIIT modes.

To carry out this upright triceps stretch, raise your arm above your head and bend at the elbow so that your hand presses against the top of your back. With your opposing hand, gently pull your elbow behind your head, feeling the hand of your stretched arm run slowly down your back.

To develop, pull further on the elbow, feeling the hand run s owly down the back.

Pectoralis Stretch

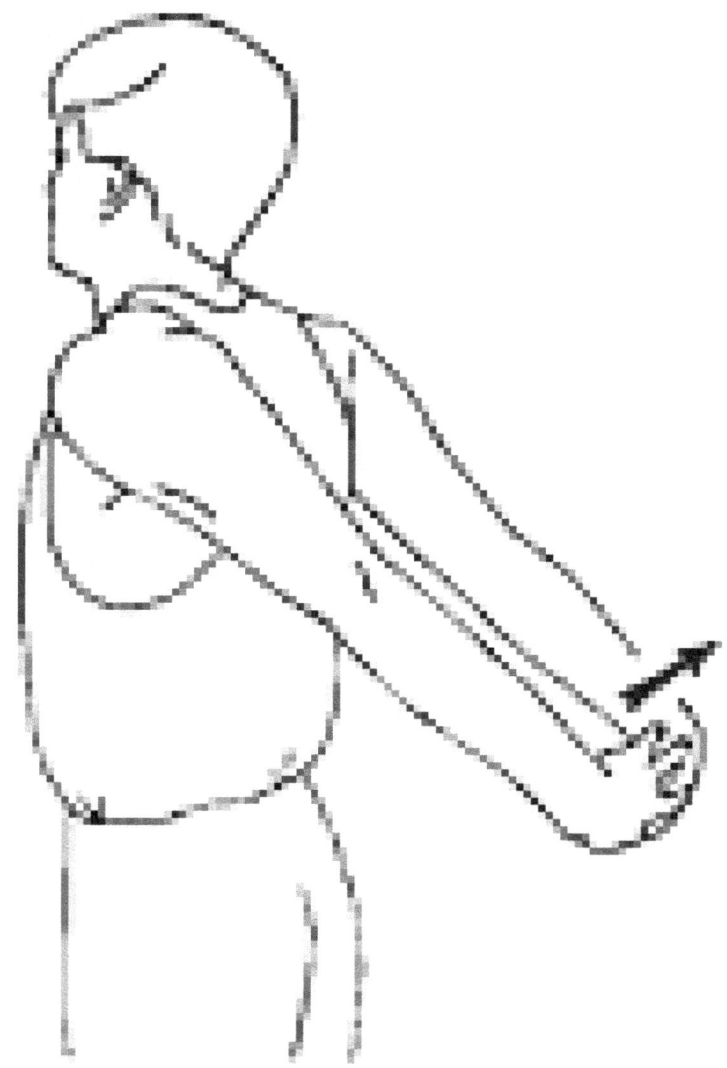

When sprinting, the upper portion of the pectorals is used to propel the arms forward, while the lower portion is used to drive them back. If you'll be carrying out sprinting yourself, which I hope you will be, then your chest will be working in overdrive. Therefore it's essential you pay attention to stretching out the pectorals, which you can do with this stretch, which also stretches the biceps.

C asp your hands behind your back and pull them away. K∃ep soft elbows while carrying out this stretch.

To develop, simply work on pulling your arms further from the body.

Advanced Pectoralis / Front Deltoids Stretch

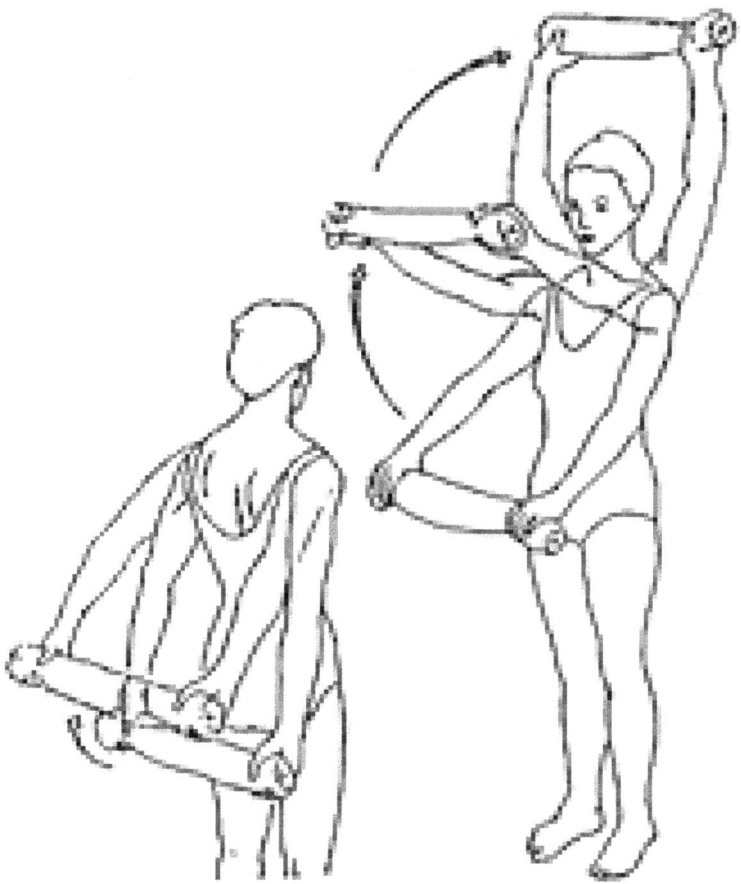

This stretch for the pectorals, front deltoids and biceps is advanced. If you stretch too deep too soon then you risk discomfort at the very least. However, this is a great stretch which you should want in your repertoire following any sprint session where the arms are used explosively.

Using a resistance band or failing that, a towel – Start with a wide grip, about one and a half shoulder widths on the towel in front of you. Raise your arms over your head and bring the towel down behind your back. When you feel the stretch – Stop. Wait until the tension wanes and then move the towel further down towards your lower back until you find a new area of tension and hold as necessary. This way you stretch both heads of the pectoralis major responsible for propulsion.

To develop further, simply narrow the grip on the towel and begin the stretch again.

Resting

There is a difference between inactivity and resting. Being inactive refers to spending your free time lying on the couch and generally being lazy. Whereas resting refers to quality time your body is using to repair, regenerate, readjust and evolve following a workout.

Resting is just as important as the workout itself as it's during the rest period that the body undergoes positive changes. And don't forget, it's during the rest stage that the magic of EPOC comes into play. It's due to EPOC that your body is still burning fat at an elevated rate for 48 hours post HIIT.

Just to clarify, by *rest* I'm not referring to the recovery periods during your HIIT session but instead to your rest days between HIIT sessions. Ideally you should carry out a HIIT session every other day, with a rest from HIIT in the days between.

I know it may be tempting to carry out two consecutive days of HIIT but I would strongly advise against it. Instead what you should do is consider your overall and longer term aims and goals. Are you on a mission to lose a lot of weight and perhaps gain muscle too? If this is the case for you, then you should incorporate HIIT sessions between strength training sessions, perhaps at your local gym. Since there's the obvious requirement for rest and recovery days between strength sessions, then having a HIIT session on your "off" days would be ideal. Strength training and HIIT utilise different physiological systems and so you can naturally work one while resting the other alternately. Although strength training is beyond the scope of this book, this author does recommend it for everybody especially if you want to lose weight - Promoting muscle growth further aids fat loss. In addition you'll benefit from an increased resting metabolism as well as increased bone, muscle, ligament and tendon strength. Indeed, whatever your goals, strength training and HIIT complement each other perfectly.

If you do undertake both a HIIT and strength training regime then it's still crucial you take a minimum of one rest day per week for recovery. Any good trainer at your gym will be able to design a training programme for you based solely on your own aims and wishes, ensuring you incorporate adequate rest days between, depending on your present fitness. In addition, you'll need to ensure you're taking in adequate nutrition to support a training regime that's this intense on the body.

If at this stage in time strength training doesn't interest you, then every second day at minimum will be a rest and recovery day. If you have the urge to take part in something active then of course there is no problem with that. However I would refrain from partaking in all-out high intensity activity and opt for something slightly more leisurely. The best thing about HIIT is that it results in superior benefits and all in the least amount of time invested – Any extra vigorous cardio activity is unnecessary.

Getting More From HIIT

We've covered all the basics including how beginners should take to their first few workouts. Now we're going to talk a little about when you become more advanced, making your HIIT workouts a little more intense in order to prevent any plateaus and to keep the weight falling off.

Following on from the last point in the above section, you may well be truly encouraged by your early progress, in fact I can assure you that this will happen. But rather than deciding to take more HIIT sessions in order to build on your progress, what I instead recommend you do is to increase the workload during your existing HIIT sessions. Remember that you will always need your rest days to maximise your gains.

You can increase your workload and make each individual H IT session more intense via the following methods:

- If your HIIT sessions are not currently stretching for a duration of 30 minutes then you can increase the number of high intensity intervals (and by default the recovery periods too), effectively making for a longer HIIT session. Remember that there's no need to extend your HIIT session to beyond 30 minutes.
- Increase the intensity of the high intensity period (if not already at 100% of your maximal heart rate).
- This should be the most important factor; decrease the duration of the recovery period, making the

entire session more intense. This should also enable you to fit in extra high intensity periods into your 30 minute session.

- Use gradients for your high intensity intervals by sprinting or cycling up hills. Increase any resistance of cardio equipment or add weights to bodyweight circuits as necessary.
- Finally, you can use one of the alternative HIIT modes as mentioned earlier to add variety and further shock your body.

Simply by phasing in these new elements over time, you'll be gradually making your HIIT session more intensive, keeping things interesting which is always recommended and you'll be exploiting your gains too.

You may have noticed that I did not add that you could "increase the length of your high intensity period." Can you guess why this is?

The reason is that if you're capable of increasing the length of your high intensity period then you're clearly not working hard enough. The aim is quality not quantity. If you're thinking to yourself that you could run for an extra five seconds at your fastest speed, then you clearly haven't been going all out at 100% up until now. The aim is to work as hard as you can, not for as long as you can - This element to HIIT is crucial.

Just to reiterate the above point and to really drill this home as it really is important; you need to set the high intensity interval period so that you really are working as hard as you're capable. The amount of time this takes is not really the issue, since if you're running, cycling or rowing as hard or as fast as you can, you will naturally fatigue within 10 – 30 seconds anyway. If you're able to sprint, cycle or row for any more than this amount of time, then you really do need to increase the intensity.

The amount of time it takes you to fatigue and require an urgent rest period will of course be different for everybody and there are many variables at play; your individual fitness, HIIT experience, which interval you're presently on, what your activity is, how you're feeling on that particular day as well as external weather conditions will al have an effect. This is why I'm very broad where I say that you'll naturally fatigue within 10 – 30 seconds. The amount of time is irrelevant as long as you do indeed work at as high an intensity as possible and you do indeed fatigue, this is all that really matters.

Conclusion

You knew when you purchased a book about losing weight that you'd be needing to do a fair amount of cardiovascular exercise. Personally I don't like classing HIIT as 'cardiovascular' exercise since it uses more than simply the cardiovascular system to supply energy to the working muscles.

If you yourself are untrained at this moment in time then I can understand that you will feel a certain amount of trepidation with regards to performing HIIT. HIIT is very intensive, which is exactly why it works so well.

You should begin very easy. Why not begin with just a couple, or three at the most, high intensity intervals and increase as you progress. I can honestly say, speaking from my experience that it is within absolutely everybody to perform activity at such high levels of exertion, so please don't be put off by HIIT. You want to lose weight fast and in the most healthy way possible and HIIT is the biggest tool at our disposal for achieving this goal.

By incorporating everything you've learned in this book, you will absolutely definitely notice improvements you never thought possible and all this with only 3 exercise sessions a week, each consisting only of around 30 minutes of your time.

Just as important as HIIT is that you also have the diet aspects correct as well, as I've explained. I promise you that if you do everything as I've set out in this book then there is no better way that has so far been discovered at helping you to lose weight, and certainly not in a way that is as fast, effective and yet as healthy as what you have learned here. Most importantly however is that the changes you make will be permanent!

Thanks once again for purchasing this book and I hope I have repaid your small investment many times over.

Now, I would like you to do two things for me; 1 – Stop reading any more weight loss material. You now know everything that you need to know in order to lose weight and by reading anymore books on this subject is merely to procrastinate. It's time to take action!

2 – Please leave an honest review on the page where you purchased this book. By doing so, you'll be helping other people in the same situation discover this book too. I read all my reviews and whether good or bad, they mean an awful lot to me and help me to improve on future works.

I wish you all the best of luck in health, fitness and life.

Also by James Driver

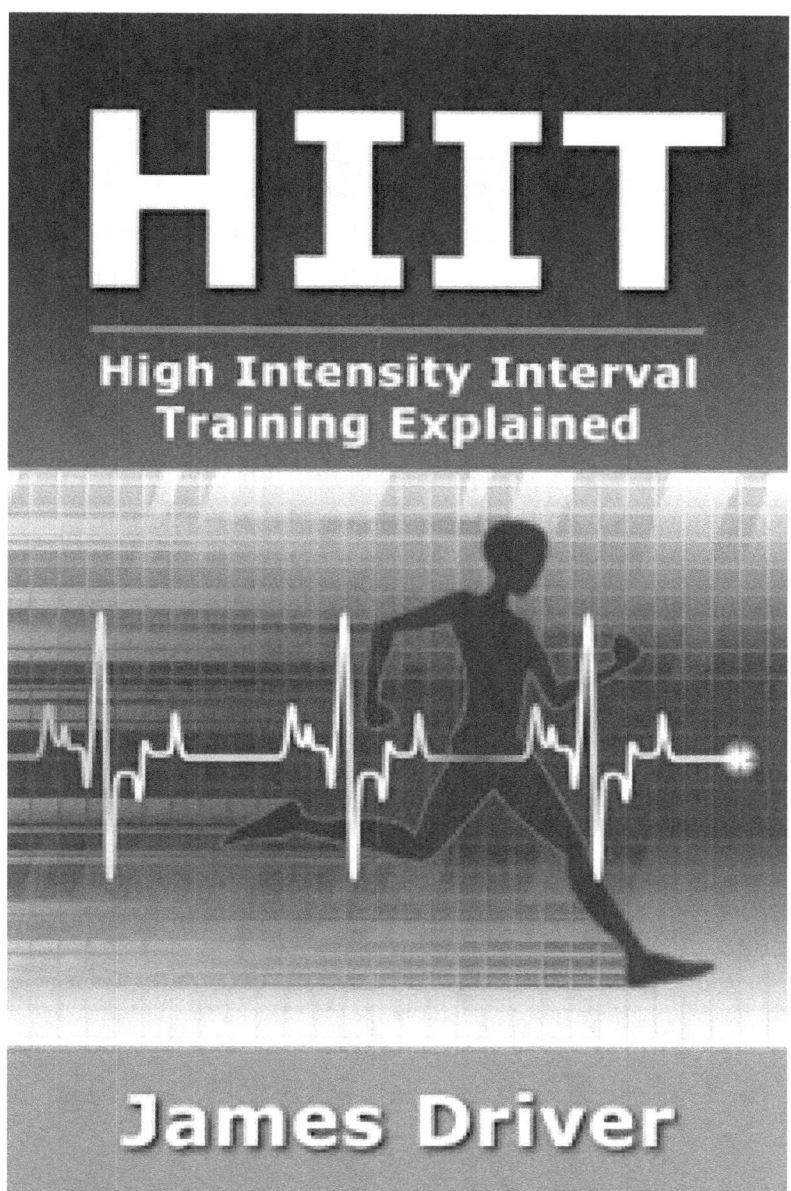

High Intensity Interval Training (HIIT) is now widely acknowledged to be the single most advantageous form of exercise for a wide range of fitness goals.

When compared side by side to other forms of cardiovascular training, HIIT repeatedly comes out on top. Not only that, but it does so in a fraction of the time when compared to continuous cardio training or steady state cardio. With HIIT, you will achieve superior gains over other forms of training in all the following areas:

- Weight loss
- Improving the body's capacity to burn fat
- Increasing the anaerobic threshold, enabling you to work harder before the burn sets in
- Improving maximal oxygen uptake (VO2 max), a popular indicator of fitness
- Improving athletic performance
- Releasing beta-endorphins, providing a feeling of well-being
- Exercise enjoyment
- And much more

H IT works by using short duration high intensity sprints together with nice and easy recovery periods such as walks or slow jogs. This makes the sprints extremely tolerable and enjoyable.

Yet few people use or even know about HIIT and its incredible power!

Find out just how effective interval training is and how it can be used in only a fraction of the time when compared to continuous training such as jogging at the same speed for up to an hour at a time.

Discover the different forms of HIIT training such as Tabata, Fartlek, the Little Method and how best to use them.

For the first time – Learn a range of high intensity exercises and training modes which are perfect for HIIT - Exercises you can perform either at the gym, in the park or at home.

Learn how to craft and make use of your own HIIT training designs, specifically to help you achieve your exercise goals in an incredibly quick time.

The science is conclusive! HIIT will change your life!

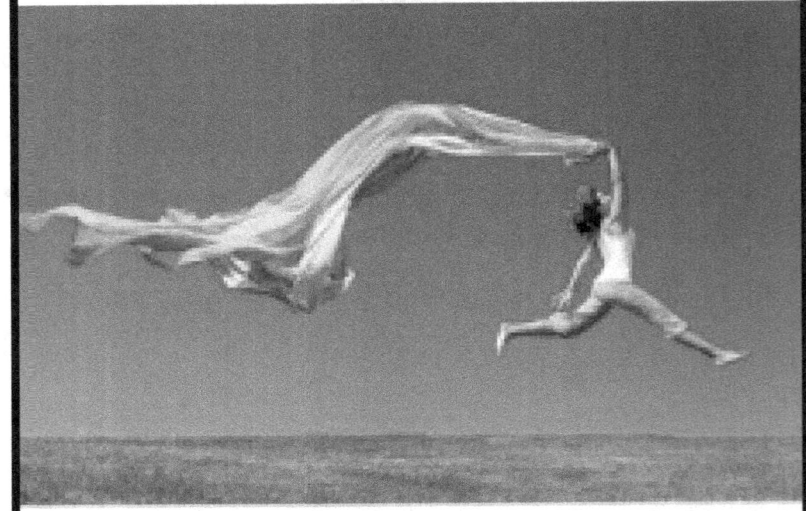

TIRED
OF FEELING
TIRED

DESTROY FATIGUE
AND RE-ENERGIZE
JAMES DRIVER

Feeling tired, lethargic or fatigued is one of the main reasons we visit the doctor. However, we are often told there's nothing wrong with us.

Chronic fatigue is the feeling of being low on energy at various points during the day for no reason whatsoever. Is this something you feel on a regular basis?

Do you struggle to pull yourself out of bed in the morning?
Do you find sleeping at night difficult?
Do you find yourself taking frequent midday naps?
Are you depressed due to your feelings of fatigue?
Are you stressed out because of this?
Are your days not as productive as they could be?
Do you pass up invitations to go out with friends due to feeling tired and fatigued?

If so then it's likely you suffer from chronic fatigue or some other condition that causes you to feel low on energy.

In this book you will discover:

- What condition, if any you may have.
- If not, then how to pin-point your lifestyle habits that are making you feel fatigued.
- Exactly what you can do to give yourself more energy than you've ever had before.

The author James Driver believes in making positive lifestyle changes that are all natural, healthy and drug free.

This is the way towards an all-round, healthy life with an abundance of energy.

T red of Feeling Tired is not full of medical language that is hard to understand and neither is it overly lengthy but is straight to the point. Tired of Feeling Tired is not for the PhD student but is instead for the individual who is suffering from this invisible condition.

Also included is a case study of a professional dancer who suffered from fatigue for many years and how she overcame it.

www.ingramcontent.com/pod-product-compliance
Lightning Source LLC
Chambersburg PA
CBHW070002_00526
45794CB0C001B/157